DICTIONARY OF
ALCOHOL USE
AND ABUSE

DICTIONARY OF ALCOHOL USE AND ABUSE

Slang, Terms, and Terminology

Compiled by Ernest L. Abel

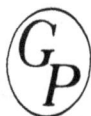

Greenwood Press
Westport, Connecticut • London, England

Library of Congress Cataloging in Publication Data

Abel, Ernest L., 1943-
   Dictionary of alcohol use and abuse.

   Bibliography: p.
   1. Alcoholism—Terminology.   2. Alcoholism—Treatment
—Terminology.   3. English language—Slang.   I. Title.
HV5017.A24   1985   362.2′92′0321   84-22521
ISBN 0-313-24631-9 (lib. bdg.)

Library of Congress Catalog Card Number: 84-22521
ISBN: 0-313-24631-9

First published in 1985

Greenwood Press
A division of Congressional Information Service, Inc.
88 Post Road West
Westport, Connecticut 06881

Printed in the United States of America

10   9   8   7   6   5   4   3   2   1

Contents

Preface

This glossary includes primarily slang terms for alcohol use and abuse in the English language, as well as some of the more common technical terms relating to the effects of alcohol and the treatment of alcohol-related problems. The names of different types of alcoholic beverages are generally omitted inasmuch as there are so many of them and they have already received separate treatment in many books. Only those beverages and mixed drinks are included here, along with a brief description of their ingredients, which are either of historical interest or are well-known representatives of particular types of beverages.

Although comprehensive, this dictionary by no means exhausts the vast lexicon of drinking. This lexicon changes so rapidly, incorporating new terms and discarding others, that any claim of comprehensiveness would be unrealistic.

Dictionary entries are arranged alphabetically, on the basis of the "something before nothing" system, for example, "B and B" and "B and S" precede "Baby." Phrases that vary by only a word, for example, "drunk as a . . . " are placed under "drunk." For other phrases, the entry is alphabetized according to the main word in the phrase, for example, "walk the chalk" is entered as "chalk, walk the."

Introduction

The precise origins of alcohol are not known. According to one version, a Babylonian creation myth, wine was a byproduct of the war between the forces of good and evil for possession of the earth. Ultimately, the forces of good triumphed but not before suffering many losses. When the good gods were slain, they fell to the earth, and from the soil in which their bodies decomposed sprang the vine, the fruit of which was the symbolic blood of the gods.

In the Biblical account, alcohol began with either Adam or Noah, depending on one's interpretation of Scripture. Those who argue that alcohol originated in the Garden of Eden do so on the basis that the forbidden fruit was the grape. But the first person whom the Bible specifically credits as planting vineyards, drinking wine, and becoming drunk was Noah.

The deliberate fermentation of both wine and beer was known in the Near East by about 3000 B.C. Wine was probably an accidental discovery, for the presence of yeast in the air naturally causes fruit juice to ferment. Beer, on the other hand, requires more than an accidental assist from nature, since air-borne yeast will not cause any significant fermentation of wort. In order to make beer, yeast must be deliberately added, and this step requires an appreciation of the forces of fermentation as well as trial and error in discovering the most appropriate strain of yeast.

The Bible notwithstanding, beer was probably produced by the Assyrians many centuries before wine. This notion is based on the fact that barley was one of the most important crops in the ancient Near East and was even the standard for trade, money being unknown until about 500 B.C. Barley was ground into flour for bread, and in the course of baking, it is theorized that someone discovered that barley mash, if treated in a certain way, could give rise to an intoxicating beverage.

In making beer, the Assyrians did not advance much beyond the preliminary stages of baking barley mash. The next stage in development occurred in Egypt where barley was allowed to germinate before making mash and brewers' yeast was added for fermentation. It was also in ancient Egypt that hops began to be added to beer to give it flavor. From the Egyptians the art of brewing passed to the Greeks and the Romans. Other civilizations independently learned the art of brewing. One area of the world in which beer-making was independently discovered was Northern Europe. In High German the beverage was called *pior* or *bior*, a term that is the origin of the present word "beer." In England, both beer (brewed with hops) and ale (brewed without hops) were popular drinks when the Anglo-Saxons invaded in the fifth century A.D.

According to another ancient myth regarding the origin of alcohol, Dionysos, the Greek god of wine, fled the ancient Near East in disgust because too much beer rather than wine was being consumed. Hence, the belief has arisen that wine was much more popular in Greece and Rome than in the Near East. From Greece, Phoenician traders transported viticulture to Spain and France. But it was in Greece and Rome that viticulture flourished and that the most critical discoveries about growing grapes and wine were made. While wine (mainly honey wine) was also consumed in England at the time of the Anglo-Saxon invasion, ale and beer remained the two main alcoholic drinks.

The next important step in making alcohol was the discovery of distillation. As long as fermentation was the only way of making alcoholic beverages, variety was limited, as was potency. (Yeast stops acting when the alcohol content reaches about 12 percent.) The discovery of distillation is attributed to an Arabian chemist, Jabir Ibn Hayyan, known to the West as Geber. Whether or not Geber himself suggested the word *al kohl* for his product, our present word "alcohol" comes from this Arabic term meaning "the essence."

While Geber may have discovered how to produce alcohol, he apparently saw little value in it. The thirteenth-century European alchemist and physician Arnoldus of Villanova, however, recognized its implications. Arnoldus probably learned the secret of distillation from the monks when he lived in Spain, and he began experimenting with the process. Since he used wine in his distilling process, his distillate was called *aqua vinae* ("water of wine"), although Arnoldus's own term was *aqua vitae* ("water of life"). Other terms by which this essence came to be known were *aqua ardens* ("strong water") and "burnt wine," which later evolved into brandy.

Initially, burnt wine was simply distilled alcohol. In the later 1500s, however, this burnt wine was added to the local wines being produced around the French town of Cognac. This "fortified" product continued to be called "burnt wine," a name that was shortened to brandy when it became the first popular wine in England and Holland during the late sixteenth century.

Not long thereafter, a Dutch professor of medicine named Fanz de le Bol (also known as Dr. Franciscus Sylvius) invented gin. Sylvius's intention was to produce a diuretic by combining juniper berries with *aqua vitae*. Instead of wine, however, he used corn and wheat grain because grain was considerably cheaper than wine. Essentially, this process amounted to distilling beer. Sylvius called his "diuretic" *genevre*, from the French word for juniper. *Genevre* attained immediate popularity among the Dutch. When English sailors docked in Holland, they, too, found it appealing and imported it to England where it was first called "geneva" and then gin.

In 1689, William of Orange, who was Dutch by birth, became King of England, and the following year, Parliament passed a law that sought to destroy the French wine trade with England, since France was Holland's trading rival. The new law was called an "Act Encouraging Distillation of Brandy and Spirits from Corn." This law revised previous laws that had been in force since the Norman Conquest, laws that prohibited the conversion of malt to distilled spirits except for medical reasons. Within four years after this law was passed, the production of distilled liquors, mainly gin, totaled about a million gallons. Within 20 years it was about 18 million gallons. In the wake of this enormous amount of drinking came an enormous amount of public drunkenness. Since anyone could legally make and sell gin, it was among the cheapest alcoholic beverages available in England, even cheaper than beer.

England was not the first country to experience public drunkenness as a social problem. Ancient Egypt also had had its problems, and admonitions against such behavior can be traced back to 1500 B.C. But it was in England that public drunkenness gave rise to a new and ever expanding vocabulary to describe the condition.

The first law in England aimed at curbing public drunkenness was passed in the sixth century by Ethelbert, the King of Kent. Other laws were passed but had little impact. Drunkenness itself became a crime in England in 1552, and in 1606 Parliament passed an act "To Repress the Odious and Loathsome Sin of Drunkenness." Various other laws were passed, but with the same result: people continued to drink to excess. Shortly after the settlement of Virginia, laws were enacted against drunkenness there too. These laws multiplied throughout the colonies, but with the introduction of rum and other distilled spirits, public drunkenness increased.

Parliament eventually became concerned about public drunkenness and passed the first Gin Act in 1729, imposing a tax on production. The law only resulted in the substitution of a low-quality product popularly called "Parliament Brandy" and was repealed in 1733. As part of the 1729 Act, a tax was placed on retail sales except when alcoholic beverages were sold in a home. Not surprisingly, about one out of every two households in London became a retail outlet. Consumption of gin became even more widespread, and gin began to replace wages for some kinds of work. Fears of general unrest caused by excessive drinking led to passage of the second Gin Act in 1736. This legislation resulted in a violent protest known as the "Gin Riots," smuggling, and a renewed popularity for beer.

In 1743, Parliament passed a third Gin Act, which imposed more moderate duties on gin and licensing of retailers. This law was replaced by yet another law, passed in 1751, after which the consumption of gin and public drunkenness finally decreased considerably.

Meanwhile, in Ireland distillers were also perfecting distillation from barley and began to produce *uisgebetha*, which eventually became known as whiskey. From Ireland, it passed into Scotland but remained primarily confined to rural districts in both countries. Irish whiskey did not become popular in London until the late 1700s. Scotch, with its characteristic blending of different kinds of whiskey, became popular a century later.

When the English colonists settled in America, they brought with them their taste for the alcoholic beverages of their homeland and the knowledge of how to produce them. Soon after settling in the New World, the colonists began distilling a new type of liquor called "kill-devil" or rum. It was first produced in Barbados from sugar cane, and the process was soon brought to New England where it became an instant favorite. Rum soon became an integral part of the Triangle Trade which involved the transport of slaves from Africa to the West Indies, and the delivery of sugar cane and molasses to New England where they were manufactured into rum.

Soon after the American Revolution, a special kind of whiskey began to be produced in Bourbon County, Kentucky. The main characteristic of this whiskey was its storage in charred-oak barrels, which caused it to lose some of its pale color and to gain a better taste. Blending techniques further refined the product. This was one of the last major developments in producing different varieties of liquor; by 1900 virtually all the different kinds of alcoholic beverages known today had been produced.

Although many influential Americans expressed negative attitudes toward the permissive and excessive use of alcohol in the New Republic, it was not until shortly after the turn of the nineteenth century that an organized effort to deal with the drinking problem began, spearheaded by the churches. Lyman Beecher, a clergyman in Litchfield, Connecticut, established the first organized temperance movement in

1813. The goal of the movement was to reduce public drinking through good example rather than through legislation. The 1830s and 1840s witnessed growing support for the temperance doctrine, as well as agitation for prohibition legislation. In 1840, the Washington Temperance Society, a forerunner of Alcoholics Anonymous, was founded, and within a few years chapters were established throughout the country. Institutions specializing in the treatment of people with alcoholic problems also began appearing in the 1840s. In 1843, the first state prohibition law was passed in the Oregon Territory, but it was revoked five years later. The first major prohibition law was passed in Maine in 1851.

With the Civil War, prohibition activities temporarily ceased, but soon thereafter prohibition efforts were renewed. In 1874, the Women's Christian Temperance Union was founded in Cleveland and placed its fight for women's rights behind the temperance movement. The first national prohibition amendment was introduced into Congress in 1876, but it was not until 1919 that national prohibition finally became law, as formulated in the Eighteenth Amendment. Although Prohibition began in the United States in 1920, no serious attempts were made to enforce it until the 1930s when speakeasies and illegal distilleries became commonplace. Already by the 1930s, opposition to Prohibition was widespread, and in 1933 it was repealed by the Twenty-first Amendment.

Pharmacological Background

Alcohol is the name of a general class of chemical compounds, but for most people, it refers to only one member of this class—ethyl alcohol, or ethanol as it is also known. Alcohol, a colorless, odorless liquid produced by fermentation, is the main constituent in alcoholic beverages. Its other main ingredients are called congeners.

The three major types of alcoholic beverages are beer, wine, and liquor. Liquors are also known as distilled spirits. Beer contains about 3 to 6 percent alcohol; wine about 10 percent (although when "fortified" with alcohol, it can contain about 20 percent); and liquor about 40 to 50 percent.

Beer is made by fermenting grains such as barley, whereas wine is made by fermenting fruit juices. Fermentation occurs as a result of the conversion of sugar into alcohol and carbon dioxide by yeast. Only about 12 percent of any material can be converted into alcohol by fermentation since at this concentration yeast activity is arrested.

Liquors such as whiskey are produced by fermenting grains as in making beer and then distilling the fermented alcohol. Because alcohol has a lower boiling point than water, it vaporizes at a lower temperature and can be separated from it and collected in a more concentrated form. Liquors are rated in terms of "proof," which means twice the percentage of alcohol. One hundred proof liquor is therefore a solution that contains 50 percent alcohol.

Alcohol is readily absorbed into the blood from the small intestine and is carried to all parts of the body. The amount of alcohol in the blood is referred to as the blood alcohol level, or blood alcohol concentration, and is given in units of gram or milligram percent of alcohol in the blood. A blood alcohol level of 0.1 percent is 0.1 grams of alcohol per 100 milliliters of blood, or 100 milligrams of alcohol in the same volume. The effects of alcohol on the body are governed by many factors, including the person's size, the amount of food eaten, if any, along with the alcohol, the rate at which alcohol is broken down into other substances (called metabolism) so that it can be eliminated from the body, a genetically determined sensitivity to alcohol, and an acquired adaptability (called tolerance) to its effects.

Americans rank about fifteenth worldwide in the amount of alcohol consumed per year, with an average per capita intake of about 2.7 gallons of absolute alcohol (pure alcohol) per adult. However, since only about two-thirds of the adult American populace drinks, the average alcohol consumption among adults who drink is about 3.9 gallons of absolute alcohol, which translates into about 1,000 cans of beer, or glasses of wine, or glasses of liquor, or any combination thereof.

The Language of Drinking and Drunkenness

The vocabulary of drinking, drunkenness, and types of alcoholic beverages is among the most extensive for any terms in the English language. If the number of words to describe a particular event or object indeed reflects the importance of that event or object to a society, then alcohol, together with its use and abuse, ranks almost supreme in the minds of the English-speaking people.

Among the basic functions of language are thought, expression, and communication. Communication on a large scale permits the coordination of group activities, and as such, language is a socializing force. It allows people to establish rapport, group identity, and solidarity; it preserves cultural traditions; and it enables culture to be transferred to subsequent generations. The need to produce an elaborate vocabulary centered around alcohol, however, has been only briefly addressed in language studies. While the vastness and richness of this vocabulary are widely recognized, the reasons for its vastness and richness have not been explicated. It does not seem to meet any of the major reasons for language development just outlined.

Perhaps one reason for the extensiveness of this language is that it is mostly slang. The essence of slang is novelty and its defiance of propriety, or what is sometimes called the "high brow." The novelty is not in the original coinage of words, but in the infusion of new meaning into already existing words. It often contains considerable humor, wit, and sarcasm, and it is usually figurative rather than literal.

A main influence on the growth of the vocabulary of drinking was the introduction of distilled beverages and the abuses that followed. The perennial desire for novelty resulted in the coining of new words and expressions for these drinks, drinking, and drunkenness. These slang terms became more and more commonplace and were coined not merely to express someone's thoughts but to distinguish the speaker by the way he or she expressed these thoughts.

Some specific slang terms tend to be associated with particular groups. In those cases, familiarity with the language identifies the user as a member of that particular group. Examples are the slang of the drug culture and the underworld. In many cases, the drug culture has adopted the slang language of alcohol (rather than vice versa). All the same, alcohol-related slang generally differs from drug slang in that very little secrecy is connected with taking alcohol and so alcohol slang does not have the same narrow "in-group" flavor. Alcohol slang, especially in slang synonyms for drunk, tends to make light of the experience, rather than hide it, and sometimes even implies a favorable attitude, for example, happy, gassed, lit. Other synonyms refer to incoordination or impairment, for example, bleary-eyed, paralyzed, tipsy. Still others suggest violence, such as kick in the guts, in the gutter, shit-faced. These differences in effects seem to reflect a general attempt at a folk-related rather than pharmacological dose-response formulation. The clearest example of such a folk-related dose-response formulation is found in the different number of "sheets in the wind," with two sheets signifying slight intoxication, three incoordination, and four or more inability to function.

The sources of slang are as varied as the scope of human activity. In general, slang seems to be playful, often incongruous. Another characteristic is economy, or what linguists call "clipping." Clipping is seen in words like "still" (which is clipped from "distilling"), and "brandy" (which is clipped from "brandy wine"). Slang in itself is of linguistic interest because it provides important insights into how language is created. No form of speech is neglected. There are metaphors (pussyfoot), metonymy (speakeasy, bootlegger), onomatopoeia (whissbang), antonomasia (Busy Bertha), hyperbole (white lightning), understatement (at rest for drunk), and irony (clear as mud).

Since vividness and novelty are the hallmarks of slang, new life is constantly being infused into older words. When usage becomes so common that a word is no longer novel, it often disappears. This is another characteristic of slang: it is very ephemeral. If these terms had not been preserved in writing, they undoubtedly would be unknown today. While most slang terms quickly become popular and just as quickly slip out of usage, many often gain public recognition and acceptance. When this happens on a large scale, these words become colloquial and eventually even standard.

Most of the words and expressions found in this glossary will likely never be anything more than slang. Nonetheless, this vocabulary, being a record of our culture's attitudes, values, reflections, and thoughts about alcohol, its use and abuse, ought to be preserved.

DICTIONARY OF
ALCOHOL USE
AND ABUSE

A

AA Alcoholics Anonymous. Self-help group of alcoholics that offers support to members trying to abstain from alcohol. Names are usually avoided to ensure anonymity.

A.A. Bum Member of Alcoholics Anonymous.

A.B.C. Alcohol Beverage Control.

About Done Drunk.

About Full Drunk.

About Gone Drunk.

About Had It Drunk.

About Right Drunk.

About Shot Drunk.

Abricotine Apricot-flavored liqueur.

Absinthe Licorice-flavored aperitif made with wormwood bark or roots and other flavorings. Now illegal in the United States, France, and several other countries because of toxicity.

Absinthism Toxic condition produced by drinking absinthe.

Absolute alcohol Pure alcohol. *See also* Alcohol.

Absorb To drink.

Abstainer One who does not drink alcoholic beverages.

Abstemious, Abstemonious Abstaining from alcohol; to be temperate or moderate in the amount of alcohol consumed.

Abstemiously Soberly.

Abstention Temperance or moderation in the amount of alcohol consumed.

Abstinence 1. Complete refraining from drinking alcoholic beverages. 2. Temperate or moderate use of alcohol.

Abstinence syndrome Withdrawal signs from chronically high level of alcohol consumption.

Abuse Alcohol consumption to the point where it results in social disapproval.

Abuser One whose drinking results in social disapproval.

A-buzz Drunk.

Accounts, Casting up his Drunk.

Aced Drunk.

Acetaldehyde Very toxic breakdown product of alcohol.

Acetate Breakdown product of acetaldehyde which can be used as energy by the body.

Acetic acid Chemical formed by bacteria causing wine to turn to vinegar.

Acetobacter The bacteria which changes wine into vinegar.

Acidity Tartness imbued by fruit acids to wine.

Acne rosacea Reddish facial appearance due to broken capillaries, caused by excessive drinking.

Acquavite *Same as* Aquavit.

Act of Parliament Beer.

Activated Drunk.

Acute Of short duration.

Acute Alcohol Poisoning Loss of consciousness and possible death due to arrest of breathing from excessive alcohol consumption.

Adam's Ale Water.

Adam's Wine Water.

Addict A compulsive drinker.

Addiction Compulsive use of alcohol. *See also* Dependence.

Addictive Having the potential to cause addiction.

Addled Drunk.

ADH Alcohol dehydrogenase.

Admiral, Tap the To drink surreptitiously.

Admiral of the Blue Tavern keeper.

Admiral of the Narrow Seas Naval term for a drunken sailor who vomits into lap of another sailor.

Admiral of the Red A drunkard.

Adrip Drunk.

Advocaat Liqueur made with eggs, brandy, and spices.

Afflicted Drunk.

Afloat Drunk.

Afloat, With Back Teeth Well *Same as* Afloat.

Afterdinner Man Heavy evening drinker.

Afternoon Man Heavy afternoon drinker.

Aftertaste Lingering taste in the mouth after wine has been swallowed.

Agardenti *Same as* Agua Ardiente.

Aging Used in reference to the "maturing" of wine or distilled spirits as they absorb the characteristics of the containers, usually wooden casks, into which they are placed.

Aglow Drunk.

Agua Ardiente, Aquadiente, Aguardiente, Aguardienta 1. Brandy distilled from red wine. 2. Any distilled liquor. 3. General term for liquor in Spanish- and Portuguese-speaking countries.

Akvavit *Same as* Aquavit.

Al K. Hol Alcohol.

Al-Anon Group name for those who are related to an alcoholic and who meet together for mutual help and support in living with an alcoholic.

Alateen Group name for teenage children of alcoholics who meet together for mutual help and support in living with an alcoholic.

Alchy, Alki, Alky 1. Liquor. 2. An alcoholic.

Alcohol Class of chemical compounds which share a particular chemical structure. More commonly used in connection with one of these compounds, ethyl alcohol, also known as ethanol or grain alcohol, a colorless liquid which is the principal intoxicating substance in wine, beer, or liquors. The concentration of alcohol in beer is about 4 percent, in table wine about 12 percent, in fortified wine about 20 percent, and in distilled spirits about 50 percent. Contrary to popular belief, alcohol is not a stimulant but a depressant. The apparent stimulant effect is due to early depression of inhibitory areas in the brain so that when these areas are depressed, an apparent stimulation occurs. In small amounts, alcohol is a euphoriant. Large amounts cause more and more depression, confusion, disorganization, loss of memory and perception, loss of coordination, and eventually loss of consciousness and death.

Alcohol abuse *See* Abuse.

Alcohol addiction *See* Addiction.

Alcohol amblyopia Damage to the optic nerve resulting in blurred vision caused by excessive drinking.

Alcohol Athlete Rumrunner.

Alcohol concentration Amount of alcohol in a specific volume of some solution. Expressed in terms of percentage volume alcohol in volume solution, e.g., 10 percent v/v, or in terms of percentage weight of alcohol in volume solution, e.g., 10 percent w/v.

Alcohol content Percentage of alcohol in a beverage.

Alcohol dehydrogenase Enzyme in the body which breaks down alcohol.

Alcohol dependence *See* Dependence.

Alcohol flush A flushed reaction to alcohol consumption, usually seen in the face. Most often occurs in Orientals and American Indians and thought to be due to higher levels of acetaldehyde. *See also* Acetaldehyde.

Alcohol poisoning Very high alcohol intake resulting in loss of consciousness.

Alcohol problems *See* Problem Drinker.

Alcohol strength *See* Proof.

Alcohol Test Test to determine how much alcohol one has consumed, usually by measuring alcohol content in breath with a Breathalyzer.

Alcoholature Alcoholic tincture.

Alcoholemia Alcohol in the blood.

Alcoholic One who is unable to decide if he should or should not drink and if he does drink is unable to stop himself. *See also* Alcoholism.

Alcoholic Amnesia *See* Blackout.

Alcoholic beverage Any potable liquid containing alcohol. There are four basic types: beer, wine, fortified wine, and distilled spirits. Each contains alcohol and water and each differs from the other in terms of percentage of alcohol ("proof") and type and quantity of congeners.

Alcoholic Beverage Control Board State agency for regulating sale and distribution of alcoholic beverages.

Alcoholic cardiomyopathy Heart disorder resulting from chronic and excessive alcohol use.

Alcoholic dementia Mental disorder resulting from chronic and excessive alcohol use.

Alcoholic disability Physical or mental problem resulting from chronic and excessive alcohol use.

Alcoholic encephalopathy Brain disorder resulting from chronic and excessive alcohol use.

Alcoholic epilepsy *See* Delirium Tremens.

Alcoholic fatty liver Abnormal fat increase in the liver caused by chronic and excessive alcohol use.

Alcoholic hepatitis Inflammation of liver and loss of liver cells caused by excessive drinking. Also associated with fatty deposits in liver.

Alcoholic paranoia *See* Delirium Tremens.

Alcoholic psychoses Mental disorder resulting from chronic and excessive alcohol use.

Alcoholic seizure *See* Delirium Tremens.

Alcoholics Anonymous (AA) Self-help organization of alcoholics founded in 1935, aimed at helping people who want to stop drinking.

Alcoholiday Drinking spree.

Alcoholism Compulsive, frequent drinking of alcohol to the point where it adversely affects the drinker's health, economic, or social situation. Medically considered as a disease characterized by inability to control drinking, leading to physical, or emotional distress.

Alcoholism Counselor Nonmedical professional who offers advice and assistance in overcoming alcohol problems.

Alcoholism Hospital Hospital specializing in treatment of alcoholism.

Alcoholist An alcoholic.

Alcoholization Producing alcohol.

Alcoholized Drunk.

Alcohologist One who studies alcohol and its effects.

Alcohology Study of alcohol-related phenomena.

Alcoholomania 1. Craving for alcohol. 2. Alcoholism.

Alcoholometer Device for measuring alcohol content in a solution by determining the solution's specific gravity.

Alcoholophilia *Same as* Alcoholomania.

Alcoholophobia Fear of alcohol.

Alcoholuria Presence of alcohol in the blood.

Aldehyde dehydrogenase Enzyme which breaks down acetaldehyde to acetic acid.

Aldehydes Congeners present in liquor, formed during the last part of the distillation process when temperature is highest. Also called feints or tails.

Ale 1. Alcoholic beverage similar to beer. Originally fermented barley made without hops. Now distinguished from beer by the specific kind of yeast used to make it which rises to the top of the ferment. Usually has higher alcoholic content than beer and a bittersweet taste. 2. Festival in England during the Middle Ages wherein ale was the main beverage consumed.

Ale Bench Bench located outside an alehouse.

Aleberry Beverage popular in England during 1600s made with boiled ale, bread, sugar, and various spices.

Alebush Bush, usually made with ivy, hung from pole outside an alehouse.

Alecie Drunkenness.

Aleconner Early government official in England who looked after quality control in ale.

Ale-dagger Dagger carried for self-protection in alehouse fights.

Ale-draper An alehouse keeper.

Ale-fed One who drinks considerable amounts of ale.

Alegar Sour ale.

Ale-garland *Same as* Alebush.

Ale-gill Ale made with ground ivy instead of hops.

Alehead A drunkard.

Alehead Wind A drunken sailor.

Alehoof *Same as* Ale-gill.

Alehorn Drinking vessel for ale made from horn of an ox or cow.

Alehouse Place where ale was served. Forerunner of the present bar.

Ale Knight One who spent a lot of time in ale houses.

Alembic Vessel used in distilling alcohol.

Alepassion Hangover.

Ale-pole *Same as* Alebush.

Ale-post *Same as* Alebush.

Ale-scop One who frequently told jokes in ale houses.

Ale-scot Tribute paid in ale.

Ale-silver Ale tax paid in London.

Ale-spinner Brewer.

Ale-stake *Same as* Alebush.

Ale-taster *Same as* Aleconner.

Ale-washed Drunk.

Alewife Woman who worked in an alehouse and usually made the ale. Forerunner of the barmaid.

Ale-wisp A drunkard.

Alight Drunk.

Al K. Hall Alcohol.

Al K. Hol Alcohol

Alk *Same as* Alchy.

Alkaloid Chemicals containing nitrogen, carbon, oxygen, and hydrogen.

Alki *Same as* Alchy.

Alki (Alky) Hall *Same as* Alchy.

Alki (Alky) Stiff 1. An alcoholic. 2. Drinker of alcohol or other inferior liquor.

Alkie Hall Alcohol.

Alkied, Alkied Up Drunk.

Alky *Same as* Alchy.

Alky-soaked Drunk.

All At Sea Drunk.

All Geezed Up Drunk.

All Gone Drunk.

All In Drunk.

All Liquored Up Drunk.

All Lit Up Drunk.

All Mops and Brooms Drunk.

All Out Drunk

All Sails Spread Drunk.

All Schnozzled Drunk.

All There Drunk.

All Wet Drunk.

Alley Juice Methyl alcohol.

Allowance A drink.

Almost Frozen Drunk.

Alpha Alcoholism Initial stage of alcoholism in which drinking has become habitual and is relied upon for relief of personal problems but has not yet impaired health.

Alt Top fermented beer. Literally "old."

Altitudes Drunkenness.

Altogethery Drunk.

Amaretto A liqueur made from apricots.

Amber Brew Beer.

Amethyst Gem believed to prevent drunkenness in ancient times.

Amethystic Preventing drunkenness.

Ammunition Alcohol.

Amontillado Dry sherry wine from Spain.

Amoroso Sweet sherry wine.

Ampelography Science of cultivating grape vines.

Amphora Vessel used in Greece and Rome to store wine so that air would be kept out.

Anchored in Sot's Bay Drunk.

Anejo Blend of rums aged for a minimum of six years.

Angel Foam Champagne.

Angel Teat Highest quality whiskey (in contrast to "bug juice," which is the lowest quality).

Angel-altogether Drunk.

Angelica Mixture of partially fermented wine, grape juice, and brandy.

Angostura Bitter flavoring sometimes added to gin.

Anis, Anisone 1. Liqueur flavored with anis. 2. Syrupy liqueur.

Anisette Sweet anis-flavored liqueur.

Another Acrobat Another drink.

Anstie's Limit About eight drinks. The amount physician Francis Anstie believed to be safe to consume on a daily basis.

Antabuse Drug used to treat alcoholism that interferes with breakdown of acetaldehyde, the metabolite of alcohol. The increased levels of acetaldehyde are so unpleasant that the alcoholic stops drinking.

Ante-Lunch Liquor taken before a meal.

Ante-Volstead Alcohol produced prior to Prohibition.

Antidry Antiprohibitionist.

Antifogmatic Any alcohol beverage.

Antifreeze 1. Alcohol. 2. Nonbeverage alcohol consumed when money for beverage alcohol is unavailable.

Antifreezed Drunk.

Anti-liquor To be opposed to the liquor business or its consumption.

Antiprohi Antiprohibitionist.

Anti-saloon League Ohio Temperance organization founded in 1893.

Antiseptic Drunk.

Anti-Tox Anti-intoxication. Drug producing sobriety in one who has been drinking a lot.

Ape Drunk Slightly intoxicated.

Aped Drunk.

Aperitif Drink taken before a meal to stimulate the appetite.

Apiculate Yeast Wild yeast found on grape skins inducing natural fermentation.

Appelation, Appelation d'Origine Term on French wine label identifying the wine's origin.

Appetizer Alcohol drink taken before meals.

Apollinaris Mineral water.

Apple Brandy *Same as* Applejack.

Applejack, Apple-jack Liquor made from apple cider.

Apple Palsy Extreme drunkenness from drinking too much Applejack.

Apple Toddy Mixed drink made with whiskey and apples.

Apple Whiskey *Same as* Applejack.

Apple Wine 1. Cider. 2. Cider to which brandy and sugar have been added and allowed to stand for about a year.

Apron Bartender.

Aqua Vitae Liquor, literally "water of life," the first term used in Europe to describe alcohol.

Aqua-duck Prohibitionist.

Aquavit Liquor distilled from potatoes and then flavored with carraway seed and cummin.

Ardent Containing alcohol.

Ardent Spirits Alcohol.

Arf and Arf Half-mixture of ale and black beer.

Arid Feeling the need for alcohol.

Arid Hound Prohibitionist.

Armagnac Type of brandy.

Aromatic wine Fortified wine flavored with herbs.

Arrack General term for liquor in Asia, Middle East, and Greece.

Asbach Type of brandy.

Asotus Drunk.

Ass on Backwards Drunk.

Astringency Oral sensation in the mouth similar to a drying sensation associated with drinking some kinds of wine.

At Ease Drunk.

At Rest Drunk.

Awakener Eye-opener; an early morning bracer.

Awash Drunk.

Awerdenty Whiskey. From Agua Ardiente.

Awry-eyed Drunk.

B

B and B Mixture of Benedictine and brandy.

B and S Brandy and Soda.

Baby 1. Newcomer at Alcoholics Anonymous. 2. Small bottle of wine or liquor, about six and a half ounces.

Baby and Nurse Small bottle containing soda water mixed with some alcohol. The baby is the bottle and the nurse is the alcohol.

Babysitter Alcoholism counsellor.

BAC Blood alcohol concentration.

Bacardi Popular brand of rum.

Bacchanal, Bacchanalia Drinking spree.

Bacchant A drunkard.

Bacchante Female drunkard.

Baccharach, Bacharach, Bachrach, Back-rag, Bachrag, Backrag Wine from the German Rhineland, very popular in the seventeenth century.

Bacchation Drunken spree. From fusion of vacation and Bacchanal.

Bacchus Bulged Drunk.

Bacchus Butted Drunk.

Baccus Wine.

Baccus, Son of A drunkard.

Back Hand Drinking more than one's share.

Back Home Drunk.

Badminton Alcohol beverage popular in England and United States during the late 1800s. Made with cucumber, sugar, nutmeg, soda water, and claret.

Bag, Put on the To drink.

Bagged Drunk.

Baked Drunk.

BAL Blood alcohol level.

Balderdash Mixture of alcoholic beverages.

Ball 1. A drink. 2. Glass of whiskey followed by a glass of beer.

Ball, On the Abstention from drinking.

Ball and a Half *Same as* Ball.

Balloon A bar.

Balloon-juice Lowerer One who abstains from drinking.

Balm Liquor.

Balm of Gilead Potent moonshine whiskey.

Balmy Drunk.

Bamboozled . Drunk.

Bane Brandy.

Bang Alcoholic content or reaction.

Bang-pitcher A drunkard.

Bang through the Elephant Drunk.

Baptized 1. Drunk. 2. Diluted alcohol.

Bar 1. Place where alcoholic beverages are sold, usually featuring a special counter or bar, behind which stands the bartender. Food is generally not served. 2. The counter behind which the bartender stands.

Bar, Over the Drunk.

Bar drinker One who drinks primarily at a bar rather than at home or at social gatherings.

Barbados Brandy Rum.

Barbados Liquor Rum.

Barbados Water Rum.

Barbecue Illegal bar.

Barfly Frequent patron of a barroom.

Barkeep, Barkeeper, Bartender One who serves drinks in a bar.

Barley Grain used in making beer.

Barley Broth, Corn, Juice, Water Beer.

Barley Cap Heavy drinker.

Barleycorn Spirits Diarrhea from excessive use of alcohol.

Barleysick Drunk.

Barleywine Beer with a high alcohol content.

Barm Froth formed at the top of fermented beer.

Barmaid Bar waitress who brings drinks to patrons.

Barman *Same as* Barkeep.

Barmy Drunk.

Barrel 1. To drink a lot of alcohol. 2. Alcoholism. 3. Standard 36 gallon container for sale of beer. *See also* Barrel sizes. 4. Container for wine. *See also* Cask.

Barrel Dosser Habitual drunkard.

Barrel Fever 1. Drunk. 2. Delirium Tremens. 3. Alcoholism.

Barrel Goods Liquor.

Barrel House 1. Bar; place where alcohol is consumed. 2. Place where the dregs from liquor barrels was sold to destitute alcoholics. 3. Speakeasy catering to a poor clientele during the Prohibition era.

Barrel House Bum Destitute drunkard.

Barrel House Drunk Very drunk, to the point of being comatose.

Barrel sizes Sizes of barrels for different volumes for beer, including: the butt (108 gallons); puncheon (72 gallons); hogshead (54 gallons); barrel (36 gallons); kilderkin (18 gallons); firkin (9 gallons); and the pin (4 1/2 gallons). All volumes are Imperial gallons. *See also* Casks.

Barrel Stiff Destitute alcoholic who supports himself by eating food from garbage cans.

Barreled (up) Drunk.

Barrique *See* Cask.

Barroom *Same as* Bar.

Bashed Drunk.

Bastard Sweet wine from Spain, popular in England during seventeenth century.

Basted Drunk

Bat, On a On a drinking spree.

Bathtub Gin Liquor illegally made by mixing alcohol with oil of juniper so that it tasted somewhat like gin.

Bats Delirium Tremens.

Batted Drunk.

Battered Drunk.

Batty Drunk.

Bay, Over the Drunk.

Bead Bubbles found around the rim of a container of moonshine whiskey after it has been shaken.

Beading oils Oil substances used to produce bubbles in moonshine whiskey so that it appears to be of better quality and higher proof than it really is.

Be-argered 1. Drunk. 2. Be-argumentative.

Bears, See the Drunk.

Beast, the Liquor.

Beat To not pay one's bar bill by walking out while the bartender is busy.

Beaujolais Fruity red wine from Beaujolais, France.

Bed Down To put to bed one who is drunk.

Been among the Philippians Drunk.

Been among the Philistines Drunk.

Been at an Indian Feast Drunk.

Been at Barbadoes Drunk.

Been at Geneva Drunk.

Been in a Storm Drunk.

Been in the Bibbing Plot Drunk.

Been in the Crown Office Drunk.

Been in the Sauce Drunk.

Been in the Sun Drunk.

Been to a Funeral Drunk.

Been to France Drunk.

Been to Jerico Drunk.

Been to Olympus Drunk.

Been to the Saltwater Drunk.

Been too Free with Sir John Strawberry Drunk.

Been with Sir John Goa Drunk.

Beer 1. Alcoholic beverage made by fermenting barley or other grains and flavored with hops. Contains between three to six percent alcohol. 2. To drink beer.

Beer, Dark Usually stout or porter, beers made by roasting malt which imparts a burnt taste and dark color.

Beer, Do a To drink a glass of beer.

Beer Baron Liquor magnate.

Beer Barrel 1. A drunkard. 2. Originally a wooden barrel lined with pitch. Now made with stainless steel or aluminum.

Beer Blast Party where large quantities of beer are consumed.

Beer-bottle One with a red face, presumably caused by excessive drinking.

Beer Bust Party where drinking beer is a major activity.

Beer can Container in which beer is sold.

Beer-eater One who drinks a lot of beer and presumably lives on beer alone.

Beer-engine Machine for raising barrels of beer from a cellar.

Beer-flip Drink similar to "egg-flip" where beer is substituted for wine.

Beer float Instrument for determining alcohol content.

Beer Garden Outdoor area next to a tavern where beer is served at tables.

Beer Gardener Proprietor of a beer garden.

Beer Hall Large indoor building in which beer is served.

Beer House Bar in which only beer is served.

Beer-jerker 1. An alcoholic. 2. A cocktail waitress. 3. One who pours beer, usually a bartender.

Beer-jugger Barmaid.

Beer life Shelf life of beer, usually about 30 days for unpasteurized beer in draft barrels and three months for bottled beer.

Beer Money Money given to English soldiers or servants instead of allowance of beer.

Beer Parlor *Same as* Beer House.

Beer preserver Device for keeping space between surface of beer and top of a barrel filled with gas to prevent spoilage.

Beer pull Handle of a Beer pump.

Beer pump Pump which raised beer in barrels located in the cellar to the bar.

Beer Saloon A bar.

Beer Shop Store where beer is sold.

Beer Slinger 1. A bartender. 2. A drunkard.

Beer Soaked Drunk.

Beer stone Calcium deposits formed during brewing on pieces of equipment.

Beerage Those whose wealth came from the sale or manufacture of beer.

Beeregar Sour beer.

Beerified Drunk; intoxicated from beer.

Beeriness Almost drunk on beer.

Beerocracy *Same as* Beerage.

Beerocrat *Same as* Beerage.

Beertorium Bar.

Beery 1. Beer-induced mellowness. 2. Undesirable smell in a bottle of wine caused by secondary fermentation in the bottle.

Befuddled Drunk.

Beginning to Fly Drunk.

Behind the Cork Drunk.

Belcher A drunkard.

Belch-guts A drunkard.

Belly Up 1. To drink at a bar. 2. Drunk.

Belly Vengeance Inferior beer.

Bellywash 1. Cheap, poor tasting liquor. 2. Nonalcoholic beverage.

Belt 1. Drink of alcohol. 2. Euphoria following alcohol consumption.

Belt the Grape To drink heavily.

Belted Intoxicated.

Bemuse To drink to the point of intoxication.

Bench Whistler A drunkard.

Bend To drink.

Bend the Elbow To drink.

Bender 1. Prolonged period of alcohol consumption. 2. A drunkard.

Bender, On a On a drinking spree.

Bending an Elbow Drinking whiskey or some other alcoholic beverage.

Bending Over Drunk.

Benedictine Type of liqueur.

Bent Drunk.

Bent an Elbow Drunk.

Bent and Broken Drunk.

Bent out of Shape Drunk.

Besot Drunk.

Besotten *Same as* Besot.

Beta alcoholism Drinking resulting in health-related problems but not dependence.

Beverage Alcohol 1. Any potable liquid containing one half a percent of alcohol or more. 2. Alcohol in beer, wine, or distilled spirits in contrast to absolute alcohol.

Bevie 1. Tavern. 2. Beer.

Bevry *Same as* Bevie.

Bewildered Drunk.

Bewitched Drunk.

Bewottled Drunk.

Beyond Salvage Drunk.

Bezzle To drink.

Bezzled Drunk.

Bezzler Heavy drinker.

B-girl Bar girl. A woman hired in a bar to induce male customers to buy drinks.

Bib To drink often. Abbreviation of bibble.

Bibacious Drunk.

Bibacity Dependent on alcohol.

Bibatory Relating to alcohol.

Bibber A drunkard.

Bibble To drink alcohol.

Bibbler *Same as* Bibber.

Bibulous Drunk.

Biffy Drunk.

Big Bottle Liquor magnate.

Big Drunk 1. A drunkard. 2. Extended drinking spree.

Big Fellow Agent of the Federal Treasury Department's Alcohol Tax Unit.

Big Head A hangover.

Big Reposer A drink before going to bed.

Biggy Drunk.

Bilberry Dram Colonial alcohol beverage made with rum and bilberries.

Biled Owl Drunk.

Bilgewater Inferior beer.

Binge Short, intense period of alcohol use.

Binge the Cask *Same as* Bull the Cask.

Bingo 1. Brandy. 2. Any liquor.

Bingo Boy An alcoholic.

Bingo Club Brandy drinkers.

Bingo Mort Female alcoholic.

Bingoed Drunk.

Birl 1. To drink with others. 2. To pay for everyone's drinks.

Bishop Popular drink during 1700s and 1800s made with hot port wine, sugar, oranges, and clove.

Bistro Wine seller or restaurant proprietor.

Bit 1. Small glass or drink of liquor. 2. Drunk.

Bit by a Fox Drunk.

Bit his Grannan Very drunk.

Bit his Name in Drunk.

Bit of Tape Liquor.

Bit of the Bottle Drink of liquor.

Bit on Slightly drunk.

Bit Teed Slightly drunk.

Bit Tiddley Slightly drunk.

Bit Tipsy Slightly drunk.

Bit Wobbly Slightly drunk.

Bite in the Brute To get drunk.

Bitten by a Barn mouse Drunk.

Bitter Diminutive of bitter beer.

Bitter Ale Ale made with more than usual amount of hops.

Bitters 1. *Same as* Bitter Ale. 2. Bitter alcoholic drink made with various herbs taken to stimulate the appetite.

Bivvy Beer.

Black-and-tan Stout and ale.

Black Betsy Whiskey.

Black-bottle Scene Barroom brawl.

Black Death Aquavit.

Black Dog Delirium Tremens.

Black Jack A large leather drinking vessel lined with pitch, used to serve beer in.

Black Pot An alcoholic.

Black Potting Fermenting mash in the still instead of a separate container.

Black Strap, Blackstrap 1. Popular, early American rum beverage mixed with molasses. 2. Very thick and sweet port wine.

Black Strap (Blackstrap) Alchy Liquor made from molasses.

Blackstrap Mollasses Dark material separated from sugar cane used to make rum.

Black Stripe Mixed drink made with rum and molasses.

Black Velvet Mixture of equal parts champagne and stout.

Blackout Period of amnesia following heavy alcohol drinking.

Blacksmith and His Helper *Same as* Boilermaker.

Blacksmith's Helper *Same as* Boilermaker.

Blanked Drunk.

Blast Rapid, strong effect from alcohol.

Blasted Drunk.

Bleary Eyed Drunk.

Bled, Drank More than He Drunk.

Blend 1. Mixture of two or more liquors or other substances. 2. Whiskey made from mixture of grains.

Blended Bourbon Whiskey Mixture of at least 51 percent straight bourbon and almost pure alcohol.

Blended Canadian Whiskey Mixture of whiskies two years old or more and distilled in Canada.

Blended Corn Whiskey Mixture of at least 51 percent straight corn whiskey and almost pure alcohol.

Blended Rye Whiskey Mixture of at least 51 percent straight rye whiskey and almost pure alcohol.

Blended Scotch Whiskey Mixture of whiskies distilled in Scotland and stored for at least three years in uncharred oak barrels.

Blewed Drunk. Variation of Blued.

Blighted Drunk.

Blimped Drunk.

Blind 1. Drunk. 2. Drinking spree.

Blind Drunk Very drunk.

Blind Pig Illegal bar.

Blind Staggers *Same as* Blind Drunk.

Blind Tiger *Same as* Blind Pig.

Blinded Drunk.

Blindo *Same as* Blind.

Blink, On a On a drinking spree.

Blink, On the Drunk.

Blinking Drunk Drunk.

Blinky Drunk.

Blissed Drunk.

Blistered Drunk.

Blithered Drunk.

Blitzed Drunk.

Bloat A drunkard.

Bloated Drunk.

Bloater A drunkard.

Block and Block Drunk.

Block and Fall 1. Cheap fortified wine. 2. Liquor. 3. Drunk and belligerent.

Blockade Whiskey.

Blockader *Same as* Runner.

Blockage Liquor.

Bloke A drunkard.

Blood Port wine.

Blood alcohol concentration, level of Amount of alcohol in the blood as a percentage of 100 milliliters of blood.

Blood and Thunder Mixture of port wine and brandy.

Blossom Nose Heavy drinker.

Blot A drunkard.

Blotter A drunkard.

Blotto Drunken unconsciousness.

Blow, Blow Out 1. Drinking spree. 2. Party where there is considerable drinking.

Blowboll A drunkard.

Blowed Drunk.

Blowing Drinking a lot.

Blown Drunk.

Blown Away *Same as* Blown.

Blown Over *Same as* Blown.

Blown Up *Same as* Blown.

Blowzy Drunk.

Blubber Foam produced when moonshine and beading oil are shaken in a bottle.

Blue Drunk.

Blue Around the Gills Drunk.

Blue Blazer Potent alcohol drink made with hot water and whiskey.

Blue Devils Delirium Tremens.

Blue-Eyed Drunk.

Blue Horrors Hallucinations associated with Delirium Tremens.

Blue Nose One who opposes the sale or use of alcohol.

Blue Pig Whiskey.

Blue Ribbon Gin.

Blue Ribbon Faker An abstainer.

Blue Ribboner *Same as* Blue Ribbon Faker.

Blue Ruin Poor gin.

Blue Stone Inferior gin.

Blue Tape Gin.

Blued Drunk.

Bluing Drinking excessively.

Bock Beer Dark, sweet beer with high alcohol content.

Bodega Place where wine is sold by the glass; a wine bar.

Body Combination of flavoring and alcoholic content in wine.

Boggled Drunk.

Boggy Drunk.

Boil To distill alcohol.

Boiled Drunk.

Boiled as an Owl Drunk.

Boiler 1. Apparatus in which mash is cooked in producing moonshine whiskey. 2. A still.

Boilermaker Drink of whiskey followed by beer.

Boilermaker's Delight Moonshine; homemade whiskey.

Boiling Drunk Drunk.

Bollixed Drunk.

Bombard Large leather flask used for liquor.

Bombard-Man One who is able to drink a lot.

Bombed Drunk.

Bombo *See* Bumbo.

Bond, In Liquor whose storage has been under government control. *See also* Bottled-in-bond.

Bonded Bourbon Straight bourbon whiskey made from corn mash and stored in government warehouse barrels for a minimum of four years. Must contain 50 percent alcohol, and is sealed with a green strip stamp provided by the U.S. Government. The product must have been produced during a single season.

Bonded Rye. *Same as* Bonded Bourbon except that grain used to produce it is rye.

Bonded Warehouse Government storage area for liquor until tax on it is paid.

Bone Prohibitionist.

Bone Dry 1. Abstinent. 2. Favoring prohibition.

Bone Dry Law Local or state prohibition law.

Boned Drunk.

Bongo, Bongoed Drunk.

Boniface's Cup Drunkenness.

Bonkers Drunk.

Boof Peach Brandy.

Boon Companion Drinking companion.

Boose *Same as* Booze.

Booster First drink in the morning.

Boosy *Same as* Boozy.

Boot Alcoholic content or reaction.

Booter Bootlegger.

Bootician High-class bootlegger.

Bootie Bootlegger.

Bootleg Illegally made liquor.

Bootlegger One who makes, sells, or distributes illegal liquor.

Booze, Bouse 1. Alcohol. 2. To drink alcohol. 3. To drink to or past the point of drunkenness.

Booze Artist An alcoholic.

Booze Baron Liquor magnate.

Booze Blind Drunk.

Booze Fencer Bartender or owner.

Booze Fest Party where a lot of alcohol is consumed.

Booze Fest, At a On a drinking spree.

Booze Fighter A drunkard.

Booze Foundry Place where liquor is made illegally.

Booze Guzzler A drunkard.

Booze Heister, Hister 1. *Same as* Bootlegger. 2. Bartender. 3. Heavy drinker.

Booze Heisting Drinking.

Booze Hitter A drunkard.

Booze Hound An alcoholic.

Booze King Heavy drinker.

Booze Legger Bootlegger.

Booze Mob Criminals who deal in alcohol.

Booze Pusher Bartender or owner.

Booze Run Trip in which liquor is smuggled.

Booze Shunter Heavy drinker.

Booze Stiff Habitual drinker.

Boozed, Boozed Up Drunk.

Boozefuddle Under the influence of alcohol.

Boozegob An alcoholic.

Boozer 1. Heavy drinker. 2. An alcoholic.

Boozery A bar.

Boozie Drunk.

Boozing Cheat Bottle of liquor.

Boozing Glass Wine glass.

Boozing Ken Tavern.

Boozy Drunk.

Borracho A drunkard.

Boskiness Drunkenness.

Bosky Drunk.

Bota Bag for wine, usually made of goatskin.

Bottle 1. Container for liquor or wine. Standard U.S. volume is one fifth of a gallon (known as 'fifth'); standard volume in England is 26.6 fluid ounces (about 1 1/3 Imperial pints). The volume of a wine bottle in England is 0.75 liters, almost identical to U.S. 'fifth.'

Bottle sizes include the magnum (double bottle), jeroboam (double magnum), rehoboam (6 bottles), methuselah (4 magnums), salamanazar (6 magnums), balthazar (8 magnums), and nebuchanezzar (10 magnums). 2. A drunkard.

Bottle Ache 1. Delirium Tremens. 2. Drunk.

Bottle-Ached Drunk.

Bottle-a-day-man A drunkard.

Bottle Ale Ale served in bottles.

Bottle Baby An alcoholic.

Bottle beer Pasteurized beer that has been carbonated and stored in bottles.

Bottle Club Private club where members can drink after legal closing hours.

Bottle Cracker A drunkard.

Bottle Drinker Member of a Bottle Gang.

Bottle Fatigue Hungover from alcohol.

Bottle Fever 1. Drunkenness. 2. Alcoholism.

Bottle Gang Group of destitute men who pool their money to buy a communal bottle of liquor or wine.

Bottle Heister A drunkard.

Bottle Man An alcoholic.

Bottle Nose Large red nose caused by heavy drinking.

Bottle Party Party at which guests bring their own liquor.

Bottle Stop Store that sells contained wine and liquor not consumed on the premises.

Bottle Sucker An alcoholic.

Bottled Drunk.

Bottled Earthquake Strong liquor.

Bottled-in-Barn *Same as* Home brew.

Bottled-in-bond Whiskey bottled at 100 proof and stored for at least four years.

Bottled Moonshine Illicit whiskey.

Bottling Works Illegal drinking place.

Bottom 1. Liquor poured in a glass to be diluted. 2. Lowest point of degradation in the life of an alcoholic associated with loss of job, family, and self-respect.

Bottom Fermentation Fermentation of grain with yeast that sinks to the bottom rather than rising to the top.

Bottom Out To experience the worst possible drinking problem before emerging and improving.

Bottomer Final drink to empty a glass.

Bottoms Dregs.

Bottoms Up Expression connected with drinking alcoholic beverages. To drain the glass or bottle.

Bounce Cherry brandy.

Bouncer Employee in a bar who evicts noisy or drunken customers.

Bouncing On a drinking spree.

Bouquet Aroma given off by wine.

Bourbon Form of whiskey made with at least 51 percent corn grain which is then aged in new charred white oak barrels. Alcohol content is 160 proof or lower.

Bourbon Poultice Whiskey.

Bouse *Same as* Booze.

Bout Drinking spree.

Bowery Bum Skid row alcoholic.

Bowl of Beer Glass of beer.

Bowsed Drunk.

Bowzed Drunk.

Bowzered Drunk.

Box-car Liquor.

Boxed Drunk.

Boxed Out *Same as* Boxed.

Bracer Drink taken to steady the nerves or to regain equanimity.

Bracer-Upper Stimulant; a pick-me-up.

Bragget, Bragot Mixture of ale, honey, and various spices boiled together and then allowed to ferment.

Brained Drunk.

Brandy Type of liquor distilled from wine or fruit mash containing about 40 percent alcohol. The type of fruit used to produce it typically precedes the name, e.g., cherry brandy. Generally aged in oak casks for 5 years.

Brandy and Fashoda Brandy and soda.

Brandy Blossom Red nose caused by excessive brandy drinking.

Brandy Face A drunkard.

Brandy Sunter Heavy brandy drinker.

Brandy-wine, Brandewine Old term for brandy.

Brannigan Prolonged drinking binge.

Brass Eye, Have a Drunk.

Brave Maker Whiskey.

Break 1. Point in the distillation process where the alcohol content begins to decrease considerably. 2. To resume drinking suddenly after a long period of abstinence.

Breaky Leg 1. Strong drink. 2. Drunkenness.

Breath alcohol Alcohol present in the breath and used to estimate amount of alcohol in the blood.

Breath Strong Enough to Carry Coal Breath from a drunk.

Breath That Will Carry Coal Breath from a drunk.

Breathalyser Instrument for measuring the amount of alcohol in the breath. This amount is then converted by the instrument into an estimate of the amount of alcohol in the blood.

Breathe a Prayer Take a drink.

Breathe Sober To avoid alcohol.

Breathing Allowing wine to stand after cork has been removed.

Breathing Sober Not drinking.

Breezy Drunk.

Brendice Large cup used for toasting someone's health.

Brew 1. To make beer or ale. 2. Beer.

Brew House Place where ale was brewed during the Early Middle Ages.

Brewer One who makes beer.

Brewer's Barm *See* Barm.

Brewer's Basket, Stole a Manchet out of Drunk.

Brewer's Grain Spent grain after fermenting and distilling, often sold as cattle feed.

Brewer's Horse A drunkard.

Brewer's Retail Government operated beer, wine, and liquor outlet.

Brewer's Yeast Type of yeast, *Saccharomyces cerevisia*, specially cultured for brewing beer.

Brewery Place where beer and ale are made.

Brewhouse *See* Brew House.

Brewmaster Person in charge of the actual brewing in a brewery.

Brick in His Hat, Got a Drunk.

Bride (Bryde) Cup Cup of wine drunk by the bride and groom at a wedding ceremony.

Bride-ale Wedding celebration at which considerable ale was served.

Bridgey Drunk.

Brigham Young Cocktail Potent whiskey.

Bright-Eyed Drunk.

Brighton Bitter Mixture of mild and bitter beer.

Bristol Cream Type of sweet sherry.

Bristol Milk Sherry.

British Champagne Porter ale.

Brix Measure of sugar content in wine.

Broach To open or "tap" a cask of wine or ale.

Broken Beer Remnants of beer.

Brook, Pissed in the Drunk.

Broth, Took his Took a drink.

Brother Bung 1. Brewer. 2. Drinking companion.

Brown ale Ale made from kiln-dried malt causing the ale to turn brown.

Brown Bag Law Local law prohibiting sale of alcohol in restaurants but which still allows customer to bring his own. Alcohol is usually brought into restaurant in a brown bag.

Brown Cow Barrel of beer.

Brown-Stone Beer.

Bruised Drunk.

Brush Whiskey Potent whiskey.

Brut Very dry, used primarily in connection with champagne.

Brut de Brut The driest of wines.

Bryde Cup *See* Bride Cup.

Bub, Bubb 1. To drink. 2. A drink.

Bubbed Drunk.

Bubber A drunkard.

Bubbing Drinking.

Bubble Water Champagne.

Bubbled Drunk.

Bubbles Champagne.

Bubbly 1. Champagne. 2. Rum.

Bucket Beer.

Bucket of Beer Bucket filled with beer.

Bucket of Blood A bar frequented by tough patrons.

Bucket of Suds *Same as* Bucket of Beer.

Bucket Shop A low-class bar.

Bucketeer Bucket shop racketeer.

Buckled Drunk.

Budge Liquor.

Budger An alcoholic.

Budgey Drunk.

Budging Ken Tavern.

Buffy Drunk.

Bug-Eyed Drunk.

Bug Hunter Thief who preys on drunks.

Bug Juice Whiskey.

Building Beer.

Bulge Drunk.

Bull Dog To place used moonshine barrels next to a burning oil drum so that the heat will sweat out whatever whiskey the barrels have absorbed.

Bull Pen Area next to a courtroom where those charged with drunkenness wait before being brought into court.

Bull the Cask To pour hot water into an empty rum barrel and let it stand so that rum will leech from the wood into the water.

Bullock's Eye A drink.

Bumbo Popular drink in Middle Ages, made with rum, sugar, water, and spices.

Bum-boozer Derelict alcoholic.

Bumclink Inferior beer.

Bummed Drunk.

Bumper Large glass of liquor filled to the brim.

Bumpsie, Bumpsy Slightly drunk.

Bumy Juice Beer.

Bun Drinking spree.

Bun, Have One On Drunk.

Bun On, Got a Drunk.

Bun-puncher Nondrinker.

Bun-strangler Nondrinker.

Bung 1. Cork in a wine cask or the removable wooden stopper in a beer barrel. 2. Bartender. 3. Owner of a tavern. 4. Brewer. 5. To serve a drink.

Bung Drawer *Same as* Bung-stave.

Bung-eyed Drunk.

Bung Hole Hole through which beer barrels are emptied and filled.

Bung Juice Beer.

Bung Starter 1. Mallet for removing the wooden bung from the bung hole. 2. Bartender.

Bung vent Hole in a barrel which allows air to enter a cask but does not allow gasses inside to escape.

Bungaree, Bungary, Bungery A bar.

Bunged Drunk.

Bungey *Same as* Bunged.

Bungfu, Bungfull Drunk.

Bung-stave Stave in a barrel for the bung hole.

Bungy Drunk.

Bunk Imitation alcohol.

Bunker Beer.

Bunned Drunk.

Buoyant Drunk.

Burdocked Drunk.

Burgundy Type of red wine originally from Burgundy, France.

Buried Drunk.

Burn with a Low (Blue) Flame Drunk.

Burned Brandy Brandy.

Burner Kerosene or gas heating unit for heating mash in making moonshine.

Burried Drunk.

Burst Drunk.

Bush Early tavern sign indicating availability of ale.

Bushhouse *Same as* Alehouse.

Business On Both Sides Of The Way Drunk.

Busky Drunk.

Bust Drinking, drinking spree.

Bust, On a On a drinking spree.

Bust Head 1. Liquor. 2. Bad whiskey.

Bust Out *Same as* Break.

Busted Drunk.

Buster One who is on a drinking spree.

Butt Large cask for wine or liquor. *See also* Cask.

Buy My Thirst Buy me a drink.

Buzz 1. Initial feelings resulting from drinking. 2. Last glass of port from a decanter.

Buzzed Slightly intoxicated.

Buzzey, Buzzy Drunk.

C

C and S Clean and sober.

Cabaret Originally a tavern. Now a restaurant where entertainment is provided along with food and drink.

Cabinet Wine German Rhine wine.

Cachaca Rum from Brazil.

Cached Drunk.

Caecuban Popular wine during the days of the Roman empire.

Caged Drunk.

Cager An alcoholic.

Calabash Liquor bottle.

Calibogus Spruce beer mixed with rum.

Calker Drink.

Call it Eight Bells Sailor's term for a drink before lunch.

Calm Scum which forms on the surface of wine stored in casks.

Calvados Apple brandy from Calvados, France.

Came Home By the Villages Drunk.

Camp Queer Place where bootleg whiskey is sold.

Campari Popular aperitif from Italy.

Can Container for moonshine whiskey, often a half-gallon fruit jar.

Can of Slop Pail of beer.

Canadian Punch Drink made with rye, rum, lemons, pineapple, and water.

Canadian whiskey Liquor similar to American whiskey except for a higher rye content and greater tendency toward blending.

Canary Light sweet wine from the Canary Islands.

Candle's-ends To drain a glass completely in a toast.

Candy Jag Craving for candy during withdrawal from alcohol.

Canned (Up) Drunk.

Canned Heat 1. Strong liquor. 2. Inferior liquor. 3. Solidified and denatured alcohol.

Canned Heater Destitute drinker who will drink anything alcoholic, including denatured alcohol.

Canon Drunk.

Canonball Swig Potent moonshine whiskey.

Can't Hit the Ground with His Hat Drunk.

Can't See Through a Ladder Very drunk.

Can't Sport a Right Light Drunk.

Can't Walk a Chalk Drunk.

Canteen Area on military post where alcohol is sold.

Canteen Medal Beer stain on clothes.

Cap Top area in a still where the vapor gathers.

Cap, Have Under His Drunk.

Cap Sick Drunk.

Capable Drunk.

Cape Horn Rainwater Rum.

Caper Juice Whiskey.

Capers, He Cuts His Drunk.

Capillaire Punch drink made with curacao, syrup, and a little water.

Capsule Protective device for corks in wine or liquor bottles.

Carafe Glass bottle with a wide base used to serve wine in restaurants.

Carboy 1. Airtight container used for fermentation. 2. A wicker-framed wine bottle.

Cardinal Popular alcohol drink in New England colonies made with oranges and red wine.

Cargoed Drunk.

Carouse 1. To have a loud and happy time. 2. Drinking spree. 3. Drinking party. 4. To drink everything given to one.

Carry It To be able to drink copiously without becoming drunk.

Carrying a Heavy Load Drunk.

Carrying a Load Drunk.

Carrying Two Red Lights Drunk.

Cart, Loaded his To have consumed alcohol to the point of intoxication.

Case Goods Bottled whiskey sold in grocery stores during the late 1890s.

Cash bar Improvised bar at a party where drinks are sold rather than provided free.

Cask Oak container for wine and liquor with various volumes including: the butt (108 gallons); the puncheon for brandy (120 gallons); the puncheon for rum (100 gallons); the pipe (115 gallons); the hogshead for rum (56 gallons); the hogshead for sherry (54 gallons); the doppleohm (65 gallons); and the barrique (50 gallons).

Cast Drunk.

Cat 1. Drunk. 2. Drunken prostitute.

Cat Lap 1. Very weak liquor. From the tendency of cats (and other animals) to avoid drinking alcohol. 2. Tea or coffee—nonalcoholic drinks.

Cat's Water Gin.

Catch Up To drink as much as those with whom one is with.

Catched Drunk.

Catsood Drunk.

Caudle Hot ale or wine drink to which spices, sugar, and other ingredients are added.

Caught Drunk.

Caulker Large and undiluted drink, usually rum or brandy.

Cawn Corn Whiskey.

Celebration Water Liquor.

Celestial Geneva Gin.

Cellar Underground area of house or warehouse where wine or liquor is stored.

Cellar, He's in the Drunk.

Cellar Smeller 1. An habitual drunkard. 2. A Government liquor enforcement officer.

Certificate of Age Certificate issued by a government stating age of a wine or liquor.

Chablis White dry wine originally from Chablis, France.

Chagrined Drunk.

Chai Aboveground wine warehouse.

Chain Lightning Bad whiskey.

Chalk Alcohol.

Chalk, Walk the Test for drunkenness in which sailors suspected of drinking were made to walk along a line drawn with chalk.

Chalybon Sweet wine from Syria consumed during Biblical era.

Champagne Type of sparkling, carbonated white wine.

Change Your Breath Invitation to drink.

Chapfallen Drunk.

Chaptalization Adding sugar or concentrated must to wine.

Char Inner burnt lining of an oak barrel that contributes to the flavor of liquor stored there.

Character Distinctive quality of a wine.

Characteristic Distinctive taste of the grape used to produce a wine.

Charge Put beer into a vat for making moonshine.

Charged Drunk.

Charring Slightly burning the inside of a liquor cask to impart flavor to the liquor it contains.

Charter the Bar To pay for everyone's drinks in a bar.

Charter the Grocery *Same as* Charter the Bar.

Chartreuse Liqueur distilled from brandy and rare herbs, produced by a religious order in France and Spain.

Chase the Duck To drink alcohol excessively.

Chaser 1. Mild drink such as beer, taken after a stronger drink, such as whiskey. 2. Alcohol taken after a nonalcoholic beverage.

Chateau Wine estate.

Cheary Drunk.

Cheer Liquor.

Cheerer Liquor.

Cheerer-Upper Drink of liquor.

Chemist One who extracts methanol from paraffin wax in canned heat by squeezing it through a handkerchief so that it can be consumed.

Cherry Bounce Colonial alcohol beverage made with rum and cherry juice.

Cherry Brandy Brandy distilled from cherry juice.

Cherry Heering Type of cherry liqueur.

Cherry Merry Mildly drunk.

Cherry Shrub *See* Shrub.

Cherubimical Drunk.

Chian Famous wine of ancient Greece.

Chianti Dry red wine from Chianti Mountains in Italy.

Chicken Whiskey Inferior whiskey.

Chickery Drunk.

Chipper Drunk.

Chips Oak chips added to moonshine to give it color and flavoring. Used to "age" moonshine more rapidly.

Chirping Glass, Taken a Consumed alcohol to the point of intoxication.

Chirping Merry Drunk.

Chloral hydrate Trichloroacetaldehyde. Sedative/hypnotic drug. When combined with alcohol it produces rapid intoxication. Combination is known as a Mickey Finn or Knockout Drops.

Choc Intoxicating alcoholic beverages.

Chocked Drunk.

Chopper, Moisten your Invitation to drink.

Christened Diluted with water.

Chronic Of long duration, as opposed to acute.

Chuck Horrors Craving for food after withdrawal from alcohol.

Chucked Drunk.

Chug-a-lug To gulp the contents of a glass until it is empty.

Churl To drink ale immediately after wine.

Cider Wine made from apple juice.

Cider Drunk Intoxicated by drinking hard cider.

Cirrhosis Liver disease associated with chronic and heavy alcohol consumption in which liver cells are replaced by scar tissue.

Citizen A nonmember of Alcoholics Anonymous.

Claret Red Bordeaux wine.

Clean-Up Periodic police efforts to remove drunks from the streets.

Clear 1. Drunk. 2. Beer after the fermented meal on top has fallen to the bottom in making moonshine.

Clear Crystal Gin.

Clear Out Drunk.

Clinched Drunk.

Clip Joint Bar that dilutes the drinks it serves or overcharges for them.

Clip the King's English To be unable to speak distinctly due to drunkenness.

Clobbered Drunk.

Closet Drinker One who drinks secretly, usually at home.

Clove Hunter An alcoholic.

Coagulated Drunk.

Coal Tar Wine.

Coarse 1. Drunk. 2. Poor quality wine.

Coast To drink steadily rather than binging to keep from going through withdrawal.

Cob Web Throat Desirous of alcohol.

Cobbler Iced wine drink to which syrup, lemon juice, and various flavors are added. Usually sipped through a straw rather than directly from the glass.

Cock-ale Drink made with ale and pieces of chicken.

Cocked Drunk.

Cocked to the Gills Drunk.

Cockeyed Drunk.

Cocktail 1. General name for any mixed drink. 2. Term used for specific mixed drinks depending on the ingredients.

Cocktail bar Bar serving cocktails as well as other drinks.

Cocktail Bum Member of Alcoholics Anonymous.

Cocktail Hour Time of day after work, usually around 5:00 to 6:00 p.m., when cocktails are served.

Cocktail stool Tall stool located next to bar in a cocktail bar.

Cod Drunkard.

Coffee Chaser Liquor taken after coffee.

Coffee Royale Coffee containing whiskey.

Coffey Still Distillation system that operates continously and produces the same quality of product regardless of where the system is located.

Cognac Brandy from Cognac, France.

Cognacked Drunk.

Coguy Drunk.

Coil Condenser in distilling moonshine.

Cointreau Liqueur made from orange peels.

Coke and Crystal Combination of cocaine and alcohol.

Coked as a Log Drunk.

Cold Drunk.

Cold Blood Beer.

Cold Cream Gin.

Cold Duck Mixture of white and red sparkling wines.

Cold Punch Mixed drink made with arrack, port wine, water, sugar, and lemon juice.

Cold Sober Sober.

Cold Tea Brandy.

Cold Turkey Abrupt abstinence from chronic drinking.

Cold Water Army Total abstainers.

Collar 1. Part of the still connecting the cap to the still. 2. Froth that forms at top of beer after it has been poured into a glass.

Color the Meerschaum To drink heavily so that one's nose becomes reddened.

Colored Drunk.

Column Still *Same as* Coffey Still.

Combo Mixed or adulterated liquor.

Comboozelated Drunk.

Comboozled Drunk.

Come Off It To stop drinking after a spree.

Come Up For Air To pass a shared bottle to the next person in a Bottle Gang.

Comform Liquor.

Comfort Liquor.

Comfortable Slightly drunk.

Comfortable Waters Liquor.

Commin' (On) Drunk.

Commissary Whiskey Whiskey ration given to soldiers in the Union Army during the Civil War.

Completely Gone Very drunk.

Completely Out Of It Drunk.

Completely Squashed Drunk.

Compo Mixed or adulterated liquor.

Compotation Party where there is considerable drinking.

Compotator Participant in a drinking party.

Concerned Drunk.

Concert-saloon Forerunner of the nightclub. Drinking place featuring entertainment and waitresses who served drinks at tables.

Concked Out Drunk.

Concoctail Cocktail.

Concord, Half Way to Drunk.

Condenser Part of a distillation apparatus where the heated alcohol vapor condenses.

Conflummoxed Drunk.

Congener Chemical substances in alcoholic beverages other than ethyl alcohol. Some are unwanted and disappear during maturation or are removed during rectification, whereas others constitute an integral part of the taste of liquors.

Connections The parts which join the various parts of a moonshiner's still.

Constitutional *Same as* Eye-opener.

Continuous Still *Same as* Coffey Still.

Controlled Drinking Drinking without becoming drunk.

Conversation Fluid Whiskey.

Conversation Water *Same as* Conversation Fluid.

Cook To reclaim denatured alcohol.

Cooked Drunk.

Cooked Liquor Mixed or adulterated liquor.

Cooker Box used to heat mash.

Cooled Tankard Popular alcohol drink in New England colonies, made with ale, white wine, and brandy.

Cooler 1. Final drink. 2. A drink at any time. 3. Alcoholic drink made with wine or whiskey, various added agents, and ice.

Cooler-off Drink of liquor.

Cooper l. Drink containing half stout and half porter. 2. Buyer or seller of illicit liquor. 3. Condenser in distilling.

Copey Drunk.

Copper 1. Pot in which mash is heated in a still. 2. Mixture of stout and porter.

Copper Nose Swollen, pimple-covered nose associated with excessive drinking.

Cop's Bottle Cheap whiskey given free by a bartender to the cop on the beat.

Coral Mickey Finn, a mixture of alcohol and chloral hydrate.

Cordial Any liqueur.

Cork Stopper for bottles made from bark of cork-oak tree.

Corkage Fee charged for opening a bottle in a restaurant, though sometimes brought by the customer himself.

Corked 1. Drunk. 2. Foul-smelling wine.

Corker Liquor.

Corkscrew Instrument for removing a cork stopper from a wine bottle.

Corkscrewed Drunk.

Corky 1. Drunk. 2. Foul-smelling wine due to a moldy cork.

Corky Wine Wine with a bad taste due to a poor cork.

Corn 1. Moonshine. 2. Whiskey made from corn.

Corn Coffee Liquor.

Corn Juice 1. Whiskey made from corn. 2. Poor quality whiskey.

Corn Likker, Liquor *Same as* Corn Whiskey.

Corn Liquor *Same as* Corn Juice.

Corn Mule Whiskey usually made from corn mash.

Corn Squeezens Moonshine.

Corn whiskey 1. Alcohol distillate made commercially and legally from corn mash which contains 80% or less alcohol. Aged in uncharred oak barrels or previously used charred oak barrels. May have a lower alcohol content than bourbon. 2. Moonshine alcohol liquor made predominantly with corn but also with sugar and possibly other grain. 3. Untaxed liquor.

Corned Drunk.

Cornered Drunk.

Corpse Reviver Potent drink of alcohol.

Corrupted Booze Diluted liquor.

Corrupted Liquor Mixed or adulterated liquor.

Councilman Alcoholism counselor.

Couple of Burning Sensations Two drinks.

Courage Liquor.

Cow Milk- or cream-based liqueur.

Cowboy Cocktail Undiluted whiskey.

Coxy-foxy Drunk.

Crack Liquor.

Crack a Bottle To drink alcohol.

Crack-Lip Prohibitionist.

Cracked Drunk.

Cracker Dry Prohibitionist.

Crackling Drunk.

Crambambull Popular alcohol drink in New England colonies; made by boiling ale, rum, and sugar.

Cramped Drunk.

Crap Dregs.

Crapula A hangover.

Crapulate To drink a large amount of alcohol.

Crapulous Drunk.

Crash Car Old car used to transport illegal whiskey and readily abandoned if the driver were in danger of arrest.

Crashed Drunk.

Crater Whiskey.

Craw Rot Inferior whiskey.

Crazed Drunk.

Crazy Drunk.

Crazy Apple Moonshine whiskey made with brandy and corn or rye whiskey.

Crazy Drunk Drunk and acting irrationally.

Crazy Water Liquor.

Cream of the Valley Gin.

Creamed Drunk.

Creature 1. Gin. 2. Any liquor.

Creature, Been Too Free With Drunk.

Creep Joint 1. Place where alcohol is sold illegally. 2. Place where alcohol is served illegally and patrons are robbed while drunk.

Creeper Joint *Same as* Creep Joint.

Creme de... Liqueur in which a particular flavor has the most noticeable taste. For example, creme de cacao has chocolate taste; creme de menthe has mint taste.

Crimson Dawn Cheap red wine.

Crock 1. An alcoholic. 2. Bottle or jug of liquor.

Crocked Drunk.

Crocko Drunk.

Crocus Drunk.

Cronk Drunk.

Crook an Elbow To take a drink.

Crooked Drunk.

Crooked Whiskey Whiskey on which government tax has not been paid.

Crooker Drunkard.

Cropsick Drunk.

Cross-eyed Drunk.

Cross-tolerance Condition in which use of one drug creates a tolerance to one or more other drugs. For example, tolerance to heroin results in tolerance to methadone; tolerance to alcohol results in tolerance to Valium and barbiturates.

Crowned Cup Cup completely filled with wine or liquor.

Crowning Office, In the Drunk.

Cru Particular vintage of wine.

Crump Drunk.

Crump Fooled Drunk.

Crumped (Out) Drunk.

Crust Solid deposit settling in bottom of bottles of red wine.

Crusta Mixed drink similar to "fancy cocktails." The rim of the glass is rubbed with lemon and then it is dipped in fine white sugar so that the sugar sticks to the edge of the glass. Other ingredients are then added.

Cry Drink of liquor.

Crying Drunk Drunk and in tears.

Crying Jag *Same as* Crying Drunk.

Cuckooed Drunk.

Cucurbit *Same as* Calabash.

Cuff Credit given by a bar for drinks.

Cup Iced wine drink to which soda water and liqueur is added.

Cup of Comfort Potent alcoholic drink.

Cup of the Creature *Same as* Cup of Comfort.

Cup That Cheers Drink of alcohol.

Cup Too Much Drunk.

Cupped Drunk.

Cups, In his Drunk.

Cupshot Drunk.

Cupshotten *Same as* Cupshot.

Curacao Liqueur made with oranges.

Currant Shrub *See* Shrub.

Curved Drunk.

Cushed Drunk.

Cut 1. Drunk. 2. To dilute liquor.

Cut Alky Diluted alcohol.

Cut Booze *Same as* Cut Alky.

Cut In the Craw Drunk.

Cut One's Throat To drink strong liquor.

Cut Throat Strong liquor.

Cutter Liquor adulterator.

Cutting Diluting the total alcohol content in distilled whiskey by adding water or some other ingredient.

Cutting House Place where alcohol was diluted and bottled, or where expensive labels were placed on bottles.

Cutting the Wolf Loose Drinking alcohol.

Cutup One on a drinking spree.

D

D and D Drunk and Disorderly.

D.O.M. Latin, *Deo Optimo Maximo* (To God Most Great); inscription placed on Benedictine labels.

Dab Small glass or drink of liquor.

Daffy 1. Gin. 2. Drunk.

Daffy's Elixir Gin.

Dagged Drunk.

Dagger Ale Strong ale.

Dago Red Cheap red wine.

Daisy General term for a mixed drink made with seltzer water.

Damage To help someone become intoxicated.

Damaged Drunk.

Damp 1. Drunk. 2. A drink.

Damp Bourbon Poultice Drink of whiskey.

Damper Liquor.

Dampish Antiprohibitionist.

Dampness Drunkenness.

Dandy Small glass of whiskey.

Dannie A drink.

Danziger Goldwasser Liqueur containing gold particles.

Daquifried Drunk.

Dark Day with Him Drunk.

Dark-brown Taste Stale mouth from drinking alcohol.

Dash 1. Small glass or drink of whiskey. 2. Mixture of wines. 3. Small amount of one type of alcoholic beverage added to another beverage.

Day Care Alcohol or drug treatment program in which patients remain at a clinic during the day and return home at night.

Daylight Space in a glass between the liquor and the top of the glass.

Dead 1. Drunk. 2. Tasteless.

Dead, On the Abstainer.

Dead Drunk *Same as* Dead.

Dead Head One who does not pay for his drinks.

Dead Man 1. Empty bottle of alcohol. 2. Drunk.

Dead Man's Dram Very potent moonshine.

Dead Marines *Same as* Dead Man.

Dead One Empty liquor bottle.

Dead Picker Robber of intoxicated persons.

Dead Soldier *Same as* Dead Man.

Dead to the World Drunk.

Deadeye Gin.

Deal a Full Hand To serve five drinks to one person.

Death Promoter Alcohol.

Debacchate To become loud and unruly as a result of drinking too much.

Debauch Drinking binge.

Debauchee A drunkard.

Debauchery Overindulgence in drinking, eating, or sex to the point of impairment.

Debbie Debutante cocktail.

Decant To pour wine from a bottle into another container so that the dregs are left behind.

Decanter Container for holding wine that has been decanted and is to be served.

Decayed Drunk.

Deck(s) Awash Drunk.

Decorate the Mahogany To treat a group to a drink.

Dee-horn, Dehorn 1. Drunkard. 2. One who drinks methyl alcohol. 3. One who drinks a lot and often begins a fight when drunk. 4. Alcohol.

Deep Cut Drunk.

Deep Drunk Very Drunk.

Defaced Drunk.

Degorgement Removal of sediment from the neck area of bottles of champagne.

Delirium Temporary state of mental disturbance with confusion, incoherence, or hallucinations.

Delirium Tremens (DTs) Psychological and physiological reactions occurring in alcoholics during drinking or withdrawal. Reactions include hallucinations, vomiting, nausea, tremor, and possibly collapse.

Delta alcoholism Inability to stop drinking. Associated with withdrawal if drinking stops.

Demi-john 1. Flask of whiskey. 2. Large glass bottle with wicker wrapping for wine.

Demon Rum Personification of the evils of alcohol consumption.

Demoralized Drunk.

Den A bar.

Denatured alcohol Alcohol to which wood alcohol has been added.

Denial Primary characteristic of alcoholism in which individual refuses to admit that he or she is dependent on alcohol.

Dependence Condition occurring as a result of continuous use of alcohol. Dependence can be either physical, psychological, or both. Physical dependence (addiction) is an adaptation of the body to the presence of a drug such that its absence precipitates a withdrawal syndrome. Psychological dependence is a condition in which the user feels a desire to continue drug use for a sense of well-being and feels discomfort when deprived of it. There is little tendency to increase the dosage in connection with psychological dependence.

Deposit Sediment that drops to the bottom of a wine container after it has been left undisturbed for some time.

Depressant Substance that dampens brain activity.

Derail Illicit liquor.

Derailed Drunk.

Dessert wine Fortified wine usually consumed after an evening meal; contains about twenty percent alcohol.

Detained on Business Drunk.

Detox, Detoxication, Detoxification Treatment program whereby an individual who is dependent on a drug is withdrawn from it under medical supervision. Symptoms associated with the withdrawal depend on the type of drug and the amount of time the individual has been using the drug. In the case of heroin dependence, the patient is gradually weaned from the drug by administering methadone; gradually reducing its dosage. In the case of alcohol dependence, Librium is often given in conjunction with withdrawal.

Detox, Detoxication, Detoxification Center Place where treatment is provided while individual undergoes detoxification.

Devil, Seen the Drunk.

Dew Drink *Same as* Eye Opener.

Dew Drop *Same as* Eye Opener.

Dew Drunk Very drunk.

Dewed Drunk.

Diastase Enzyme in malt that converts starch to sugars.

Dick Smith Private, surreptitious drink.

Diddle 1. Gin. 2. Any liquor.

Diddled Drunk.

Dido Alcohol.

Digestif After-dinner drink, usually a liqueur.

Dine-Dance-Drink-Dice-Do Drinking and gambling brothel.

Dine-Wine-Dancery Restaurant/nightclub.

Ding 1. Skid row alcoholic. 2. Drinking spree.

Ding Swizzled Drunk.

Dingbat *Same as* Ding.

Dinged Drunk.

Dingle Back room in an illegal bar.

Dingy Drunk.

Dinky Drunk.

Dionysiac Drunken revelry.

Dionysos Greek god of wine.

Dip An alcoholic. Abbreviation of Dipsomaniac.

Dipped Drunk.

Dipped His Bill *Same as* Dipped.

Dipped Too Deep *Same as* Dipped.

Dipso *Same as* Dip.

Dipsomania Craving for alcohol; alcoholism.

Dipsomaniac An alcoholic.

Dipsophobia Aversion to alcohol.

Dipsy Drunk.

Dirtfaced Drunk.

Discombobulated Drunk.

Discomboobulated Drunk.

Discouraged Drunk.

Discumfuddled Drunk.

DISCUS Distilled Spirits Council of the United States. Organization of distillers located in Washington, D.C.

Disease concept of alcoholism Concept that alcoholism is a disease in the medical sense rather than a moral problem or a form of deviant behavior.

Disguise To drink intemperately.

Disguised Drunk.

Dish, got a Drunk.

Dished Drunk.

Dishwasher Weak, inferior liquor.

Disorderly Drunk.

Dispensary System Sale of liquor through state-owned retail liquor stores.

Distillate Substance produced by distillation.

Distillation Process of separating substances in a solution by vaporization and condensation. Since alcohol vaporizes at a lower temperature than water, it will rise before water and can be recovered by condensation.

Distilled spirits Alcohol produced by distillation. In general, alcoholic beverages are first produced by heating fermented mash. Since alcohol has a lower boiling point than water, it vaporizes earlier when heated and can therefore be separated and collected. Recondensed vapor is called a distillate. The distillate thus contains a much higher concentration of pure alcohol than the initial solution.

Distiller One who produces liquor.

Distillery A bar.

Distillery Bum Skid row alcoholic.

Distillery Stiff *Same as* Distillery Bum.

Distinguished Drunk.

Disulfiram Antabuse. Drug used to help individuals stop drinking. Affects the metabolism of alcohol such that the main metabolite, acetaldehyde, accumulates in the body. Acetaldehyde causes unpleasant feelings; hence the motivation to avoid such distress is supposed to keep the individual from drinking.

Dithered Drunk.

Dithers Delirium Tremens.

Dive Place which lacks refinement where alcohol is sold.

Diving Bell Basement saloon.

Dizzify To intoxicate; make drunk.

Dizzy Drunk.

Dizzy as a Coot *Same as* Dizzy.

Dizzy as a Goose *Same as* Dizzy.

DK Drunkenness.

Do a Daniel Boone To get drunk.

Do an Edge To get drunk.

Doble-doble Beer brewed twice.

Doctor Alcohol beverage made with rum.

Doctor Hall Alcohol.

Doctor Up To add alcohol to a drink.

Doctored Adulterated.

Dodger Drink of liquor.

Dog *Same as* Bulldog.

Dog, Killed His Drunk.

Dog Drunk Very drunk.

Dog Head Large bubble that appears in the cap of a moonshiner's still.

Dog Juice Cheap wine.

Doggery 1. Illegal bar. 2. Poorly kept bar.

Doggins Reclaimed whiskey obtained from heating barrels ("bulldogging") that formerly contained the liquor.

Dog's Nose Mixture of beer and gin.

Dole-beer Beer donated by wealthy households for the poor.

Dom Perignon Well-known brand of champagne.

Domestic Liquor made in the United States.

Done a Falstaff Drunk.

Done an Archie Drunk.

Done One Right To have a drink in a "round of drinks."

Done Over Drunk.

Done Up Drunk.

Donk Home-brewed whiskey.

Dope 1. To add alcohol to a drink. 2. To adulterate alcohol.

Doped Drunk.

Doped Drink Adulterated drink.

Doped Over Drunk.

Doppleohm *See* Cask.

Dortmunder Type of German lager beer.

Dosage Sugar added to champagne before bottling.

Dose Large drink.

Dotted Drunk.

Dotty Drunk.

Double Beer.

Double Back To reuse mash in the same container to produce more moonshine.

Double Ball Four ounce glass of whiskey.

Double Beer Strong beer.

Double Geneva Gin.

Double Shot *Same as* Double Ball.

Double X Potent alcohol.

Double-Headed Drunk.

Double-Header *Same as* Double Ball.

Double-Tongued Drunk.

Doubled-Up Drunk.

Doubler Part of a distillation apparatus used to redistill previous distillates.

Doubling Redistilling moonshine whiskey to increase its alcohol content.

Doublings Redistilled product obtained from the second distillation of mash. Done by the moonshiner to increase proof strength.

Doux Very sweet, usually used in connection with wine.

Down 1. Small glass of beer. 2. Inferior beer.

Down and Out Drunk.

Down for the Count Drunk.

Down the Hatch Expression associated with drinking alcohol, meaning to pour alcohol down the throat.

Down with the Fish Drunk.

Downs Substance bar-girl drinks, usually nonalcoholic.

Draff Residue after beer or liquor have been removed from fermented malt, sometimes fed to cattle.

Draft, Draught 1. Non-carbonated beer. 2. Beer passed through filters to prevent yeast from entering bottle so that no further fermentation will occur. 3. Beer drawn from a cask instead of a bottle.

Drag Drink of liquor.

Dragging Begging for money to buy liquor.

Draggletail Drunken whore.

Dragon's Milk Strong Ale.

Drain 1. Drink of liquor. 2. Drunkard.

Drain Pipe Drunkard.

Drainist A heavy drinker.

Dram 1. A drink. 2. To take a drink.

Dram Craving To need a drink.

Dram Drinker Habitual drinker.

Dram Shop A bar.

Dram Shop Law Law which makes the owner or representative of a bar responsible for damage or injuries caused by individuals to whom he has sold alcohol.

Drambuie Oldest type of whiskey liqueur.

Dramist Heavy drinker.

Drammer Moderate drinker.

Dramster Heavy drinker.

Dranes Grain after beer has been drained from it.

Draped Drunk.

Drappin' the Bead To add concentrated alcohol to increase the proof of another beverage.

Draught, Drought 1. A drink. 2. To take a large drink of liquor all at one time.

Draught Beer *Same as* Draft.

Draw a Blank Drunk.

Draw One Down To pour a small glass of beer.

Draw One Up To pour a large glass of beer.

Dregs Sediment that remains in a barrel or glass after wine has settled.

Drench 1. To get drunk. 2. A drink.

Drench the Gizzard To drink alcohol to excess.

Drenched Drunk.

Dried Out Detoxified.

Drink 1. Any alcoholic beverage except beer. 2. To drink an alcoholic beverage.

Drink Adam's Ale To drink water.

Drink Deep To consume a lot of alcohol.

Drink-dice-dame Joint Drinking and gambling place.

Drink from the Spiggot Drink alcohol to excess.

Drink Hard *Same as* Drink Deep.

Drink Heavily *Same as* Drink Deep.

Drink Hob or Nob To drink alternately with one person and then the other.

Drink Joint A bar.

Drink like a Beast To consume a large amount of alcohol.

Drink like a Fish To consume a large amount of alcohol.

Drink Money Gratuity given to a waiter for serving drinks.

Drink One Under the Table To drink more than another drinker.

Drink One's Eyes Out *Same as* Drink Oneself Dead.

Drink Oneself Dead To Get dead drunk.

Drink Out of the Same Bottle Intimate friendship.

Drink Shop A bar.

Drink Someone under the Table To drink more than someone else in a contest to see who can drink the most alcohol.

Drinker 1. Consumer of alcoholic beverages. 2. A drunkard.

Drinkery A bar.

Drinketeria 1. Liquor establishment. 2. Cafeteria serving liquor.

Drinketorium Elaborate liquor establishment.

Drinking and Doping Carousing with liquor and drugs.

Drinking Bout Drinking spree.

Drinking House A bar.

Drinking Man Experienced consumer of alcoholic beverages.

Drinking problem Inability to control one's consumption of alcohol.

Drinkitite Liking for alcohol.

Drinkster An alcoholic.

Drive Alcohol content or reaction.

Drive Alky To smuggle liquor.

Driving under the influence (of alcohol) Impaired operation of a motor vehicle caused by drinking below the level of intoxication.

Driving While Intoxicated (DWI) Impaired operation of a motor vehicle caused by drinking at or above the level of intoxication.

Dronklew Drunken.

Drop 1. Warehouse where illegal whiskey was delivered and stored until delivered elsewhere for sale. 2. Expression current during Prohibition era. 3. A drink.

Drop, Take A To have a drink.

Drop in his Eye, Got a Drunk.

Drop of the Creature Drinking.

Drops, Took his Drunk.

Drought *Same as* Draught.

Drown the Miller Mixed or adulterated liquor.

Drown the Shamrock To drink liquor intemperately.

Drown Your Sorrows To drink alcohol excessively in order to forget what is bothering you.

Drowned Drunk.

Drugstore Liquor establishment.

Drum Place where alcohol is sold.

Drunk 1. Intoxicated. 2. One intoxicated with alcohol. 3. Drinking spree. 4. Drinking party.

Drunk, On the On a drinking spree.

Drunk and Disorderly Impaired by alcohol and behaving in a way that disrupts others.

Drunk and Irish Drunk and belligerent.

Drunk as a Badger Drunk.

Drunk as a Bastard Drunk.

Drunk as a Bat Drunk.

Drunk as a Beggar Drunk.

Drunk as a Besom Drunk.

Drunk as a Big Owl Drunk.

Drunk as a Billy Goat Drunk.

Drunk as a Boiled Owl Drunk.

Drunk as a Brewer's Fart Drunk.

Drunk as a Broom Drunk.

Drunk as a Cook Drunk.

Drunk as a Coon Drunk.

Drunk as a Coot Drunk.

Drunk as a Cunt Drunk.

Drunk as a Devil Drunk.

Drunk as a Dog Drunk.

Drunk as a Fiddler Drunk.

Drunk as a Fiddler's Bitch Drunk.

Drunk as a Fish Drunk.

Drunk as a Fly Drunk.

Drunk as a Fowl Drunk.

Drunk as a Hog Drunk.

Drunk as a Hoot Owl Drunk.

Drunk as a King Drunk.

Drunk as a Log Drunk.

Drunk as a Loon Drunk.

Drunk as a Lord Drunk.

Drunk as a Monkey Drunk.

Drunk as a Mouse Drunk.

Drunk as a Newt Drunk.

Drunk as a Nurse at a Christening Drunk.

Drunk as a Pig Drunk.

Drunk as a Piper Drunk.

Drunk as a Piss Ant Drunk.

Drunk as a Poet Drunk.

Drunk as a Polony Drunk.

Drunk as a Pope Drunk.

Drunk as a Rat Drunk.

Drunk as a Rolling Fart Drunk.

Drunk as a Sailor Drunk.

Drunk as a Skunk Drunk.

Drunk as a Soot Drunk.

Drunk as a Sow Drunk.

Drunk as a Swine Drunk.

Drunk as a Tapster Drunk.

Drunk as a Tick Drunk.

Drunk as a Wheelbarrow Drunk.

Drunk as an Owl Drunk.

Drunk as Bacchus Drunk.

Drunk as Blazes Drunk.

Drunk as Buggery Drunk.

Drunk as Chloe Drunk.

Drunk as David' Sow Drunk.

Drunk as Floey Drunk.

Drunk as Hell Drunk.

Drunk as Mice Drunk.

Drunk as the Devil Drunk.

Drunk Hole Place where destitute alcoholics can go for a meal; a mission.

Drunk in his Dumpes Drunk.

Drunk Line Line of persons arrested for public intoxication waiting to appear before the judge for sentencing.

Drunk Tank Jail where those arrested for drunkenness are kept while they await trial.

Drunkard One who regularly and willingly drinks large amounts of alcohol. A drunkard differs from an alcoholic in that he is still able to work while the latter is presumed to have no control over his drinking behavior.

Drunkard's Coat Large wooden barrel with the bottom removed and holes near the top for the head and arms. Those punished for drunkenness were required to wear it in public as a sign of disgrace during Middle Ages.

Drunkard's dyscrasia Theory of disease attributing causation to alcohol-induced changes in the blood.

Drunkard's Island Name given to Pakatoa, an island located off the coast of New Zealand, used by the Salvation Army as a place to recover from alcoholism.

Drunkard's Liver Cirrhosis.

Drunken Intoxicated.

Drunken Chalks Good conduct medal.

Drunken Horrors Delirium Tremens.

Drunkenness Intoxication.

Drunkenly Done in a drunken manner.

Drunkery A bar.

Drunkok Drunk.

Drunkometer Breathalyser.

Drunkulent Drunk.

Drunky Drunk.

Dry 1. Thirsty for a drink of alcohol. 2. Area in which alcohol is not legally sold or used. 3. Favoring prohibition. 4. Sober. 5. Wine that is not sweet.

Dry as a Gourd Favoring prohibition.

Dry Drinking Drinking without eating.

Dry Drunk Irritability occurring in an alcoholic who has not had a drink for some time.

Dry Heaves Symptom of withdrawal from alcohol, consisting of nausea and vomiting.

Drying Out Sobering up from alcohol consumption.

Drymedaries People favoring Prohibition.

Drys Individuals opposed to sale or use of alcohol.

DT-ist An alcoholic.

DTs Delirium Tremens.

Dubonnet French aperitif.

Duck 1. Liquor dealer. 2. *Same as* Bootlegger.

Due for Drydock Drunk.

Duke Gin.

Dull in the Eye *Same as* Dull-Eyed.

Dull-Eyed Drunk.

Dummy Empty liquor bottle.

Dump Low drinking place.

Dumped Drunk.

Dunk the Beak To drink liquor.

Dup the Boozing Can To enter a bar.

Dust Cutter Whiskey.

Dutch Courage Courage brought on by drinking alcohol.

Dutch Feast Party at which the host gets drunk before the guests.

Dutch Mild Beer.

Dutch Suds Beer.

Dwancery Low class drinking place.

DWI Driving while intoxicated or impaired, usually by alcohol.

Dynamite Whiskey.

Dyno Whiskey.

Dyno Joint Low drinking place.

Dyno Rouster Robber of intoxicated persons.

D'You Feel Like a Spot Invitation to drink.

E

Early Alcoholic Emerging alcoholic.

Early Purl Popular drink in England during 1800s taken soon after awakening to produce an appetite; made with hot ale, wormwood, sugar, and gin.

Ears are Ringing Drunk.

Eat and Drinkery Eating and drinking establishment.

Eau-de-vie French term for brandy. Literally "water of life."

Ebriety Drunkenness.

Ebrios Drunk.

Ebriosity *Same as* Ebriety.

Ebrious Drunk.

Ebulliometer Instrument for measuring amount of alcohol in a solution by determining boiling point of solution.

Ebullioscope *Same as* Ebulliometer.

Edge Drunkenness.

Edge On, Have an Drunk.

Edged Drunk.

Edition Drink of liquor.

Educated Thirst Having a preference for fancy mixed drinks or champagne.

Egg Nog Hot rum or brandy drink to which beaten egg is added along with various spices.

Eight, One Over the One drink too many.

Eighteenth Amendment U.S. Amendment which came into law in 1920 prohibiting manufacture, sale, and transport of alcohol, but not its consumption.

Eighteenth Amusement Eighteenth Amendment. The "Prohibition" amendment.

Eighty-six To refuse to serve any more drinks to a customer in a bar.

Elbow Bender Drunkard.

Elbow Crooker Drunkard.

Elbow Exercise Drinking.

Electrified Drunk.

Electrify To make drunk.

Elephant's Trunk Drunk.

Elevate To make drunk.

Elevated Drunk.

Elevation Drunkenness.

Elevator Liquor.

Elevener Individual who does not drink until eleven o'clock in the morning in contrast to "slingers" who drink as soon as they get up.

Eliminated Drunk

Elongated Diluted.

Embalmed Drunk.

Embalming Fluid 1. Liquor. 2. Inferior liquor.

Emperor A drunkard.

Employee Assistance Program (EAP) Occupational program to assist employees in dealing with alcoholism problems.

Emptins, Emptyings Lees of beer, cider, wine, etc.

Encephalopathy Brain damage resulting from consumption of alcohol.

English Bishop *Same as* Bishop.

Enology Study of wines.

Ensign Bearer A drunkard.

Entered Drunk.

Entire Mixture of ale, beer, and two-penny beer.

Entire Butt Beer Beer drawn from a single butt or cask.

Eonomia 1. Craving for alcohol. 2. Delirium Tremens.

Epsilon alcoholism Alcoholism characterized by binging rather than continuous drinking.

Essence of Lock Jaw Cider whiskey.

Ethanol Main alcohol in alcoholic beverages.

Ethyl alcohol *Same as* Ethanol.

Evidence Liquor.

Exalt To make drunk.

Exalted Drunk

Example, Made an Drunk.

Exchange Bar.

Excise tax Tax levied on alcohol beverages on the basis of alcohol content or quantity.

Exhilarated Drunk.

Extinguished Drunk.

Eye-Opener First drink of the day, usually early in the morning.

Eye Wash Gin.

Eye Water Gin.

F

Faced Drunk. Shit-faced.

Facer Glass of whiskey punch.

Faint Drunk.

Faithful A drunkard.

Faked Adulterated by adding more liquor.

Faker Liquor adulterator.

Falernian Popular wine during Roman Empire.

Falernum Syrup from the West Indies used to sweeten mixed drinks.

Fall To resume drinking after a period of abstinence.

Fall Off *Same as* Fall.

Fall off the Wagon *Same as* Fall.

Family Disturbance Whiskey.

Family therapy Treatment of spouse and children along with alcoholic.

Fancy Term used to describe mixed drinks in which the lip of a glass is rubbed with lemon.

Fancy Smile Drink of liquor.

Fanny A container for rum.

Fap Drunk.

Far and Near Beer.

Far Gone Drunk.

Farahead Drunk.

Farthing, Owes No Man a Drunk.

FAS Fetal Alcohol Syndrome.

Fass *See* Cask.

Fat Ale Strong ale.

Fatty liver Excessive fat accumulation in the liver associated with drinking.

Faucet Ale-house keeper.

Favorite Vice Drunkenness.

Fearless Drunk.

Featured Drunk.

Feds Agents of the Federal Treasury Department's Alcohol Tax unit.

Feel Aces Drunk.

Feel Dizzy Drunk.

Feel Frisky Drunk.

Feel Glorious Drunk.

Feel Good Drunk.

Feel Happy Drunk.

Feel His Booze Drunk.

Feel His Liquor Drunk.

Feel Juiced Up Drunk.

Feel the Effect Drunk.

Feeling No Pain Very drunk.

Feints Unwanted first and last part of distillate in making whiskey which is put aside for redistilling.

Fenian Whiskey.

Ferintosh Whiskey.

Fermentarian Drunkard.

Fermentation Chemical changes by which alcohol is produced from naturally occurring substances such as fruit juice. Fermentation usually occurs as a result of yeasts and enzymes acting on sugars.

Fermentation Engineer Distiller.

Fermentation lock Device allowing carbon dioxide to escape during fermentation without allowing air to enter.

Fermenter Container in which the mash is placed to ferment.

Fermentitian Distiller.

Fetal Alcohol Syndrome Birth defects occurring in children born to alcoholic women.

Fettered Drunk.

Fettled Ale Hot ale to which sugar, ginger, and nutmeg are added.

Feverish Drunk.

Fiddle-cup Drunk.

Fiddled Drunk.

Fiery Fluid Liquor.

Fiery Snorter Drunkard's nose.

Fiery Stuff Liquor.

Fifth Fifth of a gallon of liquor.

Fighting Drunk Quarrelsomely drunk.

Fill Up to the Bung To get very drunk.

Filling Station Liquor store.

Fine 1. To clear wine of its debris. 2. Of superior quality.

Finger 1. Small amount of alcohol. 2. *Same as* Bootlegger.

Finings Agent such as egg white used to clear suspended material from wine.

Fire Alcohol content or reaction.

Fire a Slug To take a drink of alcohol.

Fire-eater Heavy whiskey drinker.

Fire Up To Drink liquor intemperately.

Fired Up Drunk.

Firewater Liquor.

Firkin Beer barrel.

First Shot First alcohol distilled from grain.

Fishey, Fishy Drunk.

Fish-eyed, Fishy-eyed Drunk.

Fishy about the Gills Drunk.

Five-Water Grog Very diluted rum.

Fixed Drunk.

Fiz 1. Champagne. 2. Any alcohol beverage made with Apollinaris water or seltzer.

Fizzed Drunk.

Fizzical Culture Mixing drinks.

Fizzical Culturist Bartender.

Fizzled Drunk.

Flag Is Out Drunk.

Flagon Large bottle for wine.

Flake, Flakestand Container filled with cold water through which coils containing alcohol vapor pass during distillation.

Flaked Out Drunk.

Flakers Drunk.

Flakestand *Same as* Flake.

Flako Drunk.

Flannel *Same as* Yard of Flannel.

Flap Popular alcohol drink in New England colonies made with brandy and soda water.

Flap Draggon Small combustible material ignited at one end and floated in a glass of wine.

Flapper Likker Inferior liquor.

Flared Drunk.

Flash 1. Drink of liquor. 2. To vomit as a result of excessive drinking.

Flash of Lightning Glass of gin.

Flask Container for alcoholic beverages, sometimes small enough to fit into a hip pocket.

Flat Out Drunk Very drunk.

Flatch-kennurd Drunk.

Flattened Stuporous from alcohol use.

Flawed Drunk.

Flesh and Blood Brandy and Port.

Flicker To drink.

Flickering Drinking.

Flinger Person on a drinking spree.

Flip 1. Rendered unconscious by taking some drink which has been surreptitiously altered, such as a Mickey Finn. 2. Popular rum drink during the 1700s.

Float Up To get very drunk.

Floating Drunk.

Flood One's Sewers To get drunk.

Flooded Drunk.

Flooey Drunk

Flookum Powder used to make synthetic drinks.

Floored Drunk.

Floozie Older woman who frequents low-class bars.

Floppy Drunk.

Flor Type of yeast which imparts a nut-like flavor to wine.

Florid Drunk.

Florious Drunk.

Flostered Drunk.

Flowing Bowl Liquor.

Fluffy Drunk.

Flummixed 1. Confused by alcohol. 2. Drunk.

Flummoxed *Same as* Flummixed.

Flush, Flushed Drunk.

Flusher 1. Drink to rinse food down. 2. A milder drink, usually water, taken after an ardent one.

Fluster To get drunk.

Flusterate To get drunk.

Flusterated Drunk.

Flustered Drunk.

Flusticate To get drunk.

Flusticated Drunk.

Fly Blown Drunk.

Fly High To get drunk.

Flying Blind Drunk.

Flying High Drunk.

Flying Jib Talkative drunkard.

Flying Light Drunk.

Flying on One Wing Drunk.

Flying the Ensign Drunk.

Foam Beer.

Fogged Drunk.

Foggy Drunk.

Fogmatic Drunk.

Fogram Inferior liquor.

Fogrum *Same as* Fogram.

Folded Drunk.

Foolish Drunk.

Foot Bath Large glass of beer.

Forbidden Fruit Type of liqueur made with grapefruit and oranges.

Forced Down at a Hanger To be on a spree.

Foreshot First vapors that condense when alcohol beverages are made by distillation and usually discarded because of a high percentage of impurities.

Formaldehyde Inferior liquor.

Fortify To add liquor (usually brandy) to wine to increase its overall alcohol content.

Forty Rod Liquor.

Forty-Rod Lightning Strong liquor.

Forty-Two Caliber Potent liquor.

Forward Drunk.

Fossilized Drunk.

Four Bottler Drunkard.

Four Sheets in (to) the Wind Very drunk.

Four Thick Cloudy beer popular in England during the 1800s.

Four-bottle Man Drunkard.

Fox To give someone enough alcohol to make him drunk.

Fox, Caught a Very drunk.

Fox-drunk Drunk.

Foxed Drunk.

Foxhead Moonshine whiskey.

Foxiness Wine with strong grape flavor.

Foxy Drunk.

Fractured Drunk.

Frappe Drink served with finely crushed ice.

Frascati Popular Italian table wine.

Frazzled Drunk.

Free and Easy Drunk.

Freeholder Woman who accompanies her husband to a tavern.

Free-load To drink "on the house" or by having friends pay.

Free Lunch Food served without charge to those buying drinks.

Freeman's Quay To drink without paying.

Freeze One's Mouth To get drunk.

Freight Load of illicit liquor.

Freighting His Crop Drinking excessively.

French Dry vermouth.

French Article Rum.

French Cream Brandy.

French Elixir Brandy.

French Lace Brandy.

Fresh Slightly drunk.

Fresh Up To drink liquor.

Freshish *Same as* Fresh.

Fret Fermenting wine.

Fried Drunk.

Fried Egg Drunkard.

Fried On Both Sides Drunk.

Fried to the Gills *Same as* Fried.

Fried to the Hat Drunk.

Friend, Spoke with his Drunk.

Frog Eyes Large bubbles seen when the clear distillate forms in making moonshine whiskey.

Frolicate To go on a drinking spree.

Froth Beer.

Froze His Mouth Drunk.

Frozen Drunk.

Fucked Over Drunk.

Fuddle 1. To drink. 2. Drinking spree. 3. To drink to the point of intoxication.

Fuddle Cap A drunkard.

Fuddle Factory A bar.

Fuddle One's Cap To get drunk.

Fuddle One's Nose To get drunk.

Fuddle Up To drink intemperately.

Fuddled Drunk.

Fuddled as an Ape Drunk.

Fuddler Drunkard.

Fuddling Cup Drinking cup made of a number of cups fused together with a hole through each so that to empty one, all had to be emptied.

Full Drunk.

Full as a Boot *Same as* Full.

Full as a Bull *Same as* Full.

Full as a Fiddler *Same as* Full.

Full as a Goat *Same as* Full.

Full as a Goose *Same as* Full.

Full as a Lord *Same as* Full.

Full as a Tick *Same as* Full.

Full as an Egg *Same as* Full.

Full of Hops Drunk on beer.

Full-bodied High in alcohol content.

Full Cargo Drunk.

Full Cocked Drunk.

Full Flavored Drunk.

Full Hand Five large beers.

Full of Courage Drunk.

Full to the Bung Drunk.

Full to the Gills Drunk.

Full Up Drunk.

Fuller's Earth Gin.

Fully Soused Very drunk.

Fully Tanked Very drunk.

Fun Milk Liquor.

Fun Milk Parlor Elaborate bar.

Fun Water Liquor.

Funnel Heavy drinker.

Funny Drunk.

Funny Feeling Drunkenness.

Fur Brained Drunk.

Fur on his Tongue Drunk.

Furnace Source of heat under a still.

Furry Drunk.

Fusel Oil 1. Inferior liquor. 2. Congener in liquor.

Fustian Wine.

Fuzz To make drunk.

Fuzzle Factory A bar.

Fuzzled Drunk.

Fuzzy Drunk.
Fuzzy Head Drunkenness.
Fuzzy-headed Drunk.
Fuzzy Mouth Stale mouth.

G

Gaffed Drunk.

Gaga Drunk.

Gage, Gauge, Guage Cheap whiskey.

Gage, Boozed the Drunk.

Gaged Drunk

Gal Gallon.

Gall Breaker Potent alcohol beverage.

Gallon Measure of volume. 1.2 American gallons equal 1 Imperial (British) gallon. One Imperial gallon yields 6 standard British bottles of liquor. One American gallon yields 5 standard American bottles of liquor.

Gallon Distemper Delirium Tremens.

Galvanized Drunk.

Gamma alcoholism Alcoholism to the point where physical dependence has developed.

Gargle 1. Alcohol. 2. To drink alcohol.

Gargle Factory A bar.

Gargled Drunk.

Gargler Drunkard.

Gas Hound 1. An alcoholic. 2. One who drinks denatured alcohol and sterno.

Gas Load Dash of liquor.

Gas Up To drink intemperately.

Gaseous Drunk.

Gasp 1. Drink of liquor. 2. To drink.

Gassed Drunk.

Gassy Drunk.

Gatter Beer.

Gauger Government official in England who measured alcohol content in liquor to determine taxes to be paid on it.

Gawk Inexperienced bartender.

Gay Slightly drunk.

Gay and Frisky Whiskey.

Gay Lussac System Metric system for indicating strength. One hundred represents 100 percent alcohol.

Gayed Drunk.

Geared Up Drunk.

Gee 1. A drink. 2. Gallon container for alcohol. 3. Glass of liquor. 4. Liquor.

Geed, Geeded, Gheed Up Drunk.

Geesed Drunk.

Geeser 1. Drink of liquor. 2. Alcoholic. 3. Liquor glass or mug.

Geezed Drunk.

Geezer *Same as* Geeser.

Generous Drunk.

Geneva Gin.

Geneva, Been at Drunk.

Geneva Print Gin.

Gentian Predinner glass of wine.

George, Been Before Drunk.

German Conversation Water Beer.

German Goitre Beer drinker with a big belly.

Geronimo Barbiturates dissolved in alcohol.

Get a Bun On To get drunk.

Get a Dog To purchase liquor.

Get a Glow On Get drunk.

Get a Jag On To get drunk.

Get a Load On To get drunk.

Get a Shithouse On To get drunk.

Get a Skate On To get drunk.

Get a Snootful To get drunk.

Get a Thrill To get drunk.

Get an Edge on To get drunk.

Get Barreled Up To get drunk.

Get Bleary Eyed To get drunk.

Get Blotto To get drunk.

Get Boozed Up To get drunk.

Get Boozy To get drunk.

Get Bung-Eyed To get drunk.

Get Canon To get drunk.

Get Charged Up To get drunk.

Get Crocked To get drunk.

Get Cut Get drunk.

Get Dopy To get drunk.

Get Flushed To get drunk.

Get Full To get drunk.

Get Glorious Get drunk.

Get Goofy Get drunk.

Get High To get drunk.

Get It Off the Mind Drink liquor.

Get Jungled To To get drunk.

Get Light-headed To get drunk.

Get Likkered Up To get drunk.

Get Lit To get drunk.

Get Loaded To get drunk.

Get Looped To get drunk.

Get Loose To get drunk.

Get Off To stop drinking alcohol.

Get on the Band Wagon Begin drinking heavily.

Get Organized To get drunk.

Get Pickled To get drunk.

Get Right To get drunk.

Get Shot To get drunk.

Get Sloppy To get drunk.

Get Soused To get drunk.

Get Stiff To become drunk.

Get Tanked Up To get drunk.

Get the Big Head To get drunk.

Get the Gage Up To get drunk.

Get the Nose Painted Drink liquor.

Get There with Both Feet To get drunk.

Get Topsy To get drunk.

Get Up Steam Drink alcohol followed by marihuana or by intravenous injection of narcotics.

Get Warmed To get drunk.

Get Wasted To get drunk.

Get Wet To get drunk.

Get Whizzy To get drunk.

Get Woozy To get drunk.

Giddy Drunk.

Giddy Water Alcohol.

Giffed Drunk.

Giggle Champagne.

Giggle Goo Liquor.

Giggle in the Corn Corn whiskey.

Giggle Soup Liquor.

Giggle Water Champagne.

Giggled Drunk.

Gild To make drunk.

Gild Ale Ale consumed at gild meetings in Medieval England.

Gild Up To get drunk.

Gilded Drunk.

Gill 1. Drink of liquor. 2. Quarter of a pint of beer.

Gills, Blue around the Drunk.

Gills, Filled to the Very drunk.

Gills, Fishy around the Feeling the aftereffects of heavy drinking the previous day; hung over.

Gills, Green around the Drunk.

Gills, Loaded to the Very drunk.

Gin Liquor made with juniper berries or extract.

Gin and Fog Hoarseness caused by excessive drinking.

Gin Botanicals Ingredients used in making gin.

Gin Bottle Derelict alcoholic woman.

Gin Crawl Regular visits to a bar.

Gin Crazed Very drunk from consuming gin.

Gin Dive Low drinking place.

Gin Head Frequent and heavy drinker.

Gin Hound Gin drinker.

Gin Lane Moving toward drunkenness.

Gin Mill A bar.

Gin Miller Bartender.

Gin Palace Ornate saloon.

Gin-soaked Drunk from consuming gin.

Gin Spinner Gin distiller.

Gin Up To drink intemperately.

Ginger Alcohol content or reaction.

Gingered Drunk.

Ginned Drunk.

Ginnery Liquor establishment.

Ginnified Drunk on gin.

Ginny Drunk.

Ginology Drinking alcohol.

Ginters Gin-induced tremors.

Give a Bottle a Black Eye To drink liquor.

Give a Chinaman a Music Lesson To have a drink.

Give a Soldier a Black Eye To drain a bottle.

Give it a Kick To add liquor.

Give it a Wallop To add liquor.

Give Nature a Fillip To go on a drinking spree.

Give the Works To drink a cocktail.

Give Way to Booze To drink heavily and regularly.

Glace Drink chilled before serving by placing it in ice or a refrigerator, but not by putting ice into it.

Glad Drunk.

Glaized Drunk.

Glanders, Got the Drunk.

Glass, The Glass of liquor.

Glassy Drunk.

Glassy-eyed Drunk.

Glazed Drunk.

Glenlivet Famous type of Scotch.

Globular Drunk.

Glorious Drunk.

Glow 1. Initial pleasant sensation from drinking alcohol. 2. Drunkenness.

Glow On Drunkenness.

Glow Worm Frequent and heavy drinker.

Glowed Drunk.

Glowing Drunk.

Glue Liquor.

Glued Drunk.

Go 1. A drink. 2. Glass of gin.

Go behind the Scenes To get dead drunk.

Go Blind To get dead drunk.

Go Blooey To get dead drunk.

Go Dead To get dead drunk.

Go Down Drink of liquor.

Go Feed the Goldfish To have a drink.

Go Flooey To get dead drunk.

Go Haywire To get dead drunk.

Go off the Bottle To give up drinking.

Go on the Bottle Take up drinking.

Go on the Loose To go on a drinking spree.

Go on the Wagon Practice abstinence.

Go out like a Light To get dead drunk.

Go over the Cognac Trail To drink intemperately.

Go Pffft To get dead drunk.

Go Round Completed distillation.

Go See a Dog To have a drink.

Go See a Dog about a Man To have a drink.

Go See a Man about a Dog To have a drink.

Go See a Soldier/Marine To have a drink.

Go See Baby To have a drink.

Go to Bed in One's Boots To get dead drunk.

Go to the Drugstore To have a drink.

Go to Town To go on a drinking spree.

Go Under To get dead drunk.

Goa, Been with Sir John Drunk.

Goat Drunk Drunk to the point of lustfulness.

Gob Liquor smuggler.

God-awful Drunk Very drunk.

Goggled-eyed Drunk.

Goes over the Tops of Trees Drunk.

Going to Jerusalem Drunk.

Gold-headed Drunk.

Gone Drunk.

Gone a Peg too Low Drunk.

Goneness Drunkenness.

Good and Drunk Very drunk.

Good Fellow One who drinks a lot frequently.

Good Humored Drunk.

Good Luck Toast.

Good-natured Alcohol Denatured alcohol.

Good Stuff High-quality alcohol.

Goods Load of illicit liquor.

Goofy Drunk.

Googly-eyed Drunk.

Gooned, Gooned Up Drunk.

Goose, Dizzy as a Drunk.

Goose Eye Perfect bubble indicating 100 proof whiskey.

Gordon Gin.

Gordon Water Gin.

Gordoned Up Drunk on gin.

Gorey-eyed Drunk.

Got a Blow On Drunk.

Got a Brass Eye Drunk.

Got a Bun On Drunk.

Got a Buzz On Drunk.

Got a Crumb in his Beard Drunk.

Got a Dish Drunk.

Got a Drop in his Eye Drunk.

Got a Jag On Drunk.

Got a Load On Drunk.

Got a Snootful Drunk.

Got a Spur in his Head Drunk.

Got About Enough Drunk.

Got by the Head Drunk.

Got Corns in his Head Drunk.

Got his Beer on Board Drunk.

Got his Biler Loaded Drunk.

Got his Dose Drunk.

Got his Glass Eyes Drunk.

Got his Little Hat on Drunk.

Got his Nightcap on Drunk.

Got his Skinful Drunk.

Got his Tank Filled Drunk.

Got his Top Gallant Sails out Drunk.

Got More than He Can Carry Drunk.

Got on his Little Hat Drunk.

Got the Blind Staggers Drunk.

Got the Glanders Drunk.

Got the Gout Drunk.

Got the Horns On Drunk.

Got the Indian Vapors Drunk.

Got the Nightmare Drunk.

Got the Pole Evil Drunk.

Gout, Got the Drunk.

Government Alcohol Alcohol bought from a Prohibition officer.

Gowed Drunk.

Gowed to the Gills Very drunk.

Grab a Snort To drink liquor.

Grace Cup Large communal tankard, usually made of silver, with two to four handles.

Grain neutral spirits Almost pure alcohol produced by distilling grain mash. Contains over 190 proof.

Grain spirits Alcohol distilled from fermented grain mash and aged in oak casks. As a result of storage the alcohol acquires certain qualities not contained in grain neutral spirits.

Grand Marnier French liqueur made from oranges.

Granny Fee Bribe money paid to law-enforcement officers to keep them from interfering with moonshine production.

Grape Wine.

Grape Bloom Waxy covering on grapes.

Grape Monger Wine drinker.

Grape Must Fresh grape juice.

Grape Shot, Grapeshot Drunk on wine.

Grape Sugars Sugars in grapes which are easily fermented.

Grappa Brandy made from leftover grape skins.

Grapple-the-rails Whiskey.

Grappo, Grapo 1. Fruitmash whiskey. 2. Wine.

Grasshopper Medication for treating alcohol intoxication.

Graveled Drunk.

Grease Spot Place where bribes were paid so that moonshine could be transported to various towns.

Grease the Gills To drink liquor.

Greased Drunk.

Greased Lightning Strong liquor.

Green Guts One unaccustomed to liquor.

Green Goods Alcoholic beverages.

Green Grocery Grocery store that also sold alcohol on the premises.

Green Liquor Raw moonshine.

Grenadine Syrup used making mixed drinks.

Grey Paste Neurological symptoms of chronic alcohol usage.

Gripe Waters Liquor.

Groatable Drunk.

Grocery A bar.

Grog 1. Diluted rum. 2. General term for distilled liquor. 3. To drink hard liquor.

Grog, Have Grog on Board To be slightly drunk.

Grog Blossom Facial pimple or blotch caused by drinking too much grog.

Grog Fight Drinking session.

Grog Hound An alcoholic.

Grog Merchant Saloon owner.

Grog on board Drunk.

Grog Shop A bar.

Grog Tub Bottle of brandy.

Grog Up To drink intemperately.

Grogged, Grogged Up *Same as* Groggy.

Groggery Seedy drinking place.

Groggified *Same as* Groggy.

Grogging Diluting.

Groggy 1. Drunk. 2. Unsteady on one's feet due to too much alcohol.

Groove, In the Abstaining from alcohol.

Grotable *Same as* Groatable.

Growler of Beer Pitcher, pail, or other container for beer.

Guard One who watches out for Treasury agents and gives warning to moonshiners.

Guinea Red Cheap Italian wine.

Gulch A drunkard.

Gullet Wash Liquor.

Gulsh Dregs from wine or beer.

Gum Tickler Strong drink.

Gumption Apple brandy.

Gunnels, Loaded to the Drunk.

Gunpowder Proofing Using gunpowder to test for proof. *See also* Proof.

Gurgle Liquor.

Gussey Drunkard.

Gut Full To have consumed enough to make one drunk.

Gut Warmer Liquor.

Guts Alcoholic content or reaction.

Guts, Kicked in the Drunk.

Gutter, In the Drunk.

Guttered Drunk.

Guttle To take a drink.
Guyed Out Drunk.
Guzzle To drink large amounts of alcohol.
Guzzle Guts Drunkard.
Guzzled Drunk.
Guzzler An alcoholic.
Guzzling Drinking.
Guzzlery A bar.

H

Habitual 1. Chronic; on a regular basis. 2. Chronic drunkard.

Habituation Psychological, in contrast to physiological, dependence. Characterized by a desire rather than a craving for drug use based on a feeling of well-being associated with such use. Does not involve tolerance or serious medical complications upon withdrawal. Deleterious effects mainly involve the individual rather than society. The term is now rarely used because of the difficulty in distinguishing it from dependence.

Had a Couple of Drinks Slightly Drunk.

Had a Cup Too Much *Same as* Had Enough.

Had a Dram Drunk.

Had a Few Too Many Drunk.

Had a Little Drunk.

Had a Little Too Many Drunk.

Had a Snort Drunk.

Had Enough Consumed alcohol to the point of intoxication.

Had his Cold Tea Drunk.

Had One or Two Drunk.

Hail-Fellow-All-Wet One who is drunk.

Haily Gaily Slightly Drunk.

Hair of the Dog that Bit You Alcohol taken as a remedy for a hangover the morning after a drinking spree.

Hair on his Tongue Drunk.

Hair Raiser Strong drink of liquor.

Half Small glass of beer.

Half a Brewer Drunk.

Half a Load On Drunk.

Half and Half Mixture of two brewed substances such as beer and stout.

Half Bent Out of Shape Drunk.

Half in the Bag Drunk.

Half in the Boot Drunk.

Half the Bay Over Drunk.

Half the Bay Under Drunk.

Half Under Drunk.

Half Up the Pole Drunk.

Half-assed Drunk.

Half-barreled Drunk.

Half-blind Drunk.

Half-bulled Drunk.

Half-canned Drunk.

Half-cocked Drunk.

Half-corked Drunk.

Half-corned Drunk.

Half-crocked Drunk.

Half-cut Drunk.

Half-geared Drunk.

Half-gone Drunk.

Half-goofed Drunk.

Half-jacked Drunk.

Half-lit Drunk.

Half-loaded Drunk.

Half-looped Drunk.

Half-mocus Drunk.

Half-muled Drunk.

Half-on Drunk.

Half-out Drunk.

Half-pickled Drunk.

Half-pissed Drunk.

Half-rats Drunk.

Half-rinsed Drunk.

Half-screwed Drunk.

Half-seas over Drunk.

Half-shaved Drunk.

Half-shot Drunk.

Half-slewed Drunk.

Half-snapped Drunk.

Half-sober Drunk.

Half-soused Drunk.

Half-sprung Drunk.

Half-stewed Drunk.

Half-stiff Drunk.

Half-tanked Drunk.

Half-tipsy Drunk.

Halfway house Care facility for homeless alcoholics serving as interim home between detoxication and independence.

Halfway to Concord Drunk.

Hall Alcohol.

Hallelujah Syrup Whiskey.

Hammer To beg for money to be used for buying alcohol.

Hammered Drunk.

Hammerish Drunk.

Hammock, Slewed in his Drunk.

Hanced Drunk.

Handle One's Liquor To remain sober.

Hang One On To drink alcohol to the point of intoxication.

Hangar Liquor establishment.

Hangover Distress experienced after drinking alcohol the day before. Usually consists of splitting headache made worse by loud noises and bright light, dizziness, malaise, heartburn, loss of appetite, nausea, and vomiting.

Hangover Breakfast Late breakfast after a drinking spree.

Hangover Monday Monday after a weekend drinking spree.

Happy Slightly Drunk.

Happy as a King *Same as* Happy.

Happy Hour Unspecified time after work when drinks are served at a reduced price.

Happy Wet Stout or porter ale.

Harbor Beer Very weak beer.

Hard Case Case of liquor.

Hard Cider Cider that has fermented.

Hard drinker One who drinks a lot.

Hard liquor Any liquor, in contrast to beer or wine.

Hard Stuff *Same as* Hard Liquor.

Hard Water Liquor.

Hardware Load of illicit liquor.

Hardy Drunk.

Has a Bag On Drunk.

Has a Big Head Headache from drinking.

Has a Brass Eye Drunk.

Has a Brew To have a beer.

Has a Brick in One's Hat Drunk.

Has a Bun On Drunk.

Has a Can on Drunk.

Has a Drink To have a drink of alcohol.

Has a Drive Containing alcohol.

Has a Drop in his Eye Drunk.

Has a Full Cargo Drunk.

Has a Gargle To drink liquor.

Has a Glow On Slightly Drunk.

Has a Guest in the Attic Drunk.

Has a Head On Experiencing a hangover.

Has a Jag On Drunk.

Has a Kick Containing alcohol.

Has a Load On Drunk.

Has a Noggin On Headache from drinking.

Has a Package On Slightly Drunk.

Has a Pinch of Snuff in his Wig Drunk.

Has a Quiet One To drink by oneself.

Has a Rubber Drink Experiencing a hangover.

Has a Shine On Drunk.

Has a Skate On Drunk.

Has a Slant On Drunk.

Has a Snoot Full Drunk.

Has a Time Go on a drinking spree.

Has an Edge On Drunk.

Has Business on Both Sides of the Way Drunk.

Has Cast Iron Guts To be able to drink anything.

Has his Back Teeth Well Afloat Drunk.

Has his Flag Out Drunk.

Has his Gage Up Drunk.

Has his Head on Backwards Drunk.

Has his Pots On Drunk.

Has his Wet Sheet Aboard Drunk.

Has One on Me Have a drink and I will pay for it.

Has One's Spot Hit To drink liquor.

Has One's Swill To drink liquor intemperately.

Has Taken Hippocrates' Grand Elixir Drunk.

Has the Heeby-jeebies Drunk.

Has the Jumps Experiencing a hangover.

Has the Screaming Meemies Drunk.

Has the Whoops and Jingles Drunk.

Has the Zings Drunk.

Hat, Got on his Little Drunk.

Haunted with Evil Spirits Drunk.

Hazy Drunk.

He Man Cocktail Potent cocktail.

Head Froth on the surface of beer that has been quickly poured into a glass.

Head, Got by the Drunk.

Head Full of Bees Drunkenness.

Headache 1. Cocktail. 2. Liquor.

Heads and Tails Distillate obtained at the beginning and end of the distillation process; contains a high amount of unwanted congeners.

Heady 1. Drunk. 2. Having a high alcohol content.

Health, Drink his To offer a toast.

Hearing the Owl Hoot Becoming Drunk.

Heart's Ease Gin.

Hearty Liquor.

Heated his Copper Drunk.

Heater and Cooler Large beer taken after a small glass of liquor.

Heavy Having a very high alcohol content.

Heavy drinking 1. Drinking more than some social norm. 2. Consumption of some specific amount as designated by some arbitrary criterion, e.g., two or more drinks a day.

Heavy Wet Malt liquor.

Hedge Tavern.

Hedge-hog Quills Drink of cider.

Heeby Jeebies Delirium Tremens.

Heel *Same as* Heeltaps.

Heel Kicker-Upper One on a drinking spree.

Heeled Drunk.

Heels a Little Slightly Drunk.

Heels and Sets *Same as* Heels a Little.

Heeltaps Liquor left in the bottom of a glass.

Hefty Strong liquor.

Heimgemacht Beer.

Hell Around Go on a drinking spree.

Hell Raising On a drinking spree.

Hellbender Drinking spree.

Helpless Drunk.

Helpless Drunk Alcoholic totally unable to care for himself.

Here's at You Toast.

Here's Blowing the Lid Toast.

Here's Cheeri-Oh Toast.

Here's Cheers Toast.

Here's Down the Alley Toast.

Here's Fortune Toast.

Here's God Bless Us Toast.

Here's Good Luck Toast.

Here's Hearts and Flowers Toast.

Here's How Toast.

Here's Into Your Face Toast.

Here's Jolly Good Luck Toast.

Here's Looking At You Toast.

Here's Looking to You Toast.

Here's Mud in Your Eye Toast.

Here's Pie in Your Face Toast.

Here's Something in Your Eye Toast.

Here's the Best Toast.

Here's the Best of Luck Toast.

Here's the Hatch Toast.

Here's the Rat Hole Toast.

Here's the Rat Trap Toast.

Here's the very Best Toast.

Here's to Absent Friends Toast.

Here's to You Toast.

Het Up Drunk.

Hey-Heyer One on a drinking spree.

Hiccius-doccius Drunk.

Hiccough Drink of liquor.

Hiccus Drunk.

Hickey Slightly Drunk.

Hiddey Drunk.

Hi-De-Ho Drinking spree.

High 1. Slightly Drunk. 2. Euphoric from alcohol.

High and Light Mildly drunk.

High as a Fiddler Drunk.

High as a Georgia Pine Drunk.

High as a Kite Drunk.

High as Lindbergh Drunk.

High as the Sky Drunk.

Highball Iced drink usually made with whiskey and soda.

High-bottom A.A. Member of Alcoholics Anonymous who has not yet completely faced up to his problem.

High-geared Strong liquor.

High Go Drinking spree or party.

High Goer One on a drinking spree.

High Jinks 1. Drinking spree. 2. Dice game to see who pays for drinks at a bar.

High license system Policy of charging owners of saloons a large annual tax in order to regulate the number of saloons.

High Lonesome Drunk.

High-Powered Strong liquor.

High-Pressure Salesmanship Strong liquor.

High Shots *Same as* High Wines.

High-toned Tonic Liquor.

High up to Picking Cotton Slightly Drunk.

High Voltage Strong liquor.

High Wines Purer alcoholic distillation resulting from distilling whiskey twice. Usually containing about 70 to 80 percent pure alcohol.

Highball Mixed drink served in a tall glass.

Higher than a Kite Drunk.

Highsiding *Same as* High.

Hijacker Robber of a bootlegger.

Hilts, Loose in the Drunk.

Hip Flask Small flask of liquor that fits into a hip pocket.

Hipped Drunk.

Hippocras Mixture of wine and honey, popular in England during 1500s–1600s.

Hippocrates' Grand Elixir Liquor.

Hippocrates' Sleeve Filter through which Hippocras was poured to separate undissolved matter.

H'ist One To have a drink.

Hister A heavy drinker.

Hit a Soldier Drink from the bottle.

Hit Bottom *See* Hitting Bottom.

Hit by a Barnmouse Drunk.

Hit it up To go on a drinking spree.

Hit the Booze *Same as* Hit the Bottle.

Hit the Bottle Drinking heavily on a regular basis to the point of intoxication.

Hit the Hooch *Same as* Hit the Bottle.

Hit the Jug *Same as* Hit the Bottle.

Hit the Pots *Same as* Hit the Bottle.

Hit the Sauce *Same as* Hit the Bottle.

Hit the Skids To be losing all of one's savings and family due to excessive use of alcohol.

Hit the Wine *Same as* Hit the Bottle.

Hitting Bottom Total personal disaster caused by drinking, including impaired health, loss of job, breakdown of family, and loss of self-respect.

Hoary eyed Drunk.

Hob or Nob? Invitation to drink.

Hock Wine from German Rheinland.

Hocky, Hockey Drunk.

Hocus To place a drug into wine or some other alcoholic beverage to induce stupefaction so that the consumer can be robbed.

Hocus Pocus Drunk.

Hog Drunk Very Drunk.

Hog Wash Beer.

Hogshead Barrel for storing wine or beer.

Hoist One To drink an alcoholic beverage.

Hoister Drunkard.

Hol Alcohol.

Hold One's Liquor Ability to drink without becoming intoxicated.

Hold Over Hangover.

Hold-out Artist Skid-row alcoholic who does not share his supply with others.

Hollands Gin.

Hollow Leg Ability to consume a considerable amount of alcohol without becoming drunk, as if the alcohol were being poured into a hollow leg.

Home, Knows not the Way Drunk.

Home Town Bum *Same as* Homeguard.

Homebrew Alcoholic beverage made in the home.

Homebrewery Homebrew still.

Homeguard Skid-row alcoholic who remains in the city in which he was born.

Homespun Alcohol.

Honey Dip Liquor.

Honked Drunk.

Honky-tonk Saloon with a low class clientele.

Hooch, Hootch 1. Alcohol. 2. Bootleg whiskey.

Hooch Fest Drinking spree or party.

Hooch Graft Liquor Business.

Hooch Hister Heavy drinker.

Hooch Hound Drunkard.

Hooch House Liquor establishment.

Hooch Humps Low spirits after drinking.

Hooch Up To intoxicate; make drunk.

Hooched Drunk.

Hoocher An alcoholic.

Hoocherie Liquor establishment.

Hoodman Very Drunk.

Hook Drink of liquor.

Hooker Large drink of liquor.

Hoop Mark placed on a drinking cup to indicate quantity consumed.

Hoop it Up Drinking spree.

Hooping up Drinking spree.

Hootch *Same as* Hooch.

Hootcher *Same as* Hoocher.

Hooted Drunk.

Hop Toad Potent alcoholic beverage.

Hop Up Intoxicate, Make Drunk.

Hopped, Hopped Up Drunk.

Hopfest Drinking party.

Hopping Hipped Quarrelsomely Drunk.

Hops Dried flowers of the hops plant which are added to beer to give it a characteristic bitter taste.

Horizontal Drunk.

Horn A drink.

Hornson, Got the Drunk.

Horny Man Federal Treasury Alcohol Tax Unit agent.

Horrors Delirium Tremens.

Horse Blanket Whiskey Whiskey made in a crude still using a blanket to collect the distillate.

Horseback Drunk.

Hosed Drunk.

Hot 1. Drunk. 2. Liquor.

Hot as a Red Wagon Drunk.

Hot Bottle Liquor bottle.

Hot Boozle Liquor bottle.

Hot Flash Strong drink of liquor.

Hot Pot Ale and brandy boiled together.

Hot Stuff Liquor.

Hot Toddy Mixture of whiskey and hot black coffee.

Hot Water Liquor.

Hotcha-Brew Liquor.

Hot-headed Drunk.

Hotter than a Boiled Owl Quarrelsomely Drunk.

Hotter than a Skunk Very Drunk.

Hound Drunkard.

How About a Stop? Invitation to drink.

How-come-ye-so Drunk.

How'll You Have It? Invitation to drink.

How's About a Little Moisture Invitation to drink.

Huff Cap Strong ale.

Hum Very strong ale made by adding liquor.

Humid Glass of beer.

Hummer Drinking spree.

Humming Potent, extra strong ale.

Humpty Dumpty Ale boiled with brandy.

Hung One On Consumed enough alcohol to have become considerably drunk.

Hunter's Hoop *Same as* Hoop.

Hush House Illicit liquor establishment.

Hush Shop *Same as* Hush House.

Hushie *Same as* Hush House.

Hydromel *Same as* Mead.

Hydrometer Instrument for measuring the amount of sugar in wort.

I

I subscribe Statement made before drinking.

Ice Palace Elaborate bar.

ID Card Identification Card, a document showing the possessor's age so that he may purchase alcoholic beverages legally.

Ignite Oil Whiskey.

Ignorant Oil Wine.

Ill-Natured Alcohol Denatured alcohol.

Illuminate To intoxicate.

Illuminated Drunk.

Illusion Distortion in perception of a stimulus, in contrast to an hallucination which has no basis in external stimulation.

I'm with you Statement made before taking a drink.

Imbibed too much Drunk.

Imbibery A bar.

Imperial *Same as* Methuselah.

Impotence Decrease or absence of a male's ability to function sexually, or a decrease or absence in fertility.

In a Fix Drunk.

In a Fog Drunk.

In a Fuddle Drunk.

In a Muddle Drunk.

In a Stew Drunk.

In a Trance Drunk.

In Armor Quarrelsomely drunk.

In Beer Drunk.

In Color Drunk.

In Drink Drunk.

In for It Drunk.

In his Airs Drunk.

In his Ales Drunk.

In his Altitudes Drunk.

In his Armor Drunk.

In his Beer Drunk.

In his Cups Drunk.

In his Element Drunk.

In his Glory Drunk.

In his Pots Drunk.

In his Prosperity Drunk.

In Liquor Drunk.

In Orbit Drunk.

In the Bag Drunk.

In the Cellar Drunk.

In the Clouds Drunk.

In the Gutter Drunk.

In the Pen Drunk.

In the Pink Drunk.

In the Pulpit Drunk.

In the Rats Drunk.

In the Sack Drunk.

In the Satchel Drunk.

In the Suds Drunk on beer.

In the Sun Drunk.

In the Tank Drunk.

In the Wind Drunk.

In Uncharted Waters Drunk.

In vitro Outside the body. Generally refers to chemical reactions occurring in test tubes, flasks, etc.

In vivo Inside the body. Generally refers to chemical reactions occurring in the body.

Incognito Drunk.

Indian Liquor Cheap whiskey sold to Indians.

Indian Whiskey *Same as* Indian Liquor.

Indisposed Drunk.

Indoor Tan Red complexion caused by drinking.

Inebriant Drunkard.

Inebriate 1. Drunk. 2. A drunkard.

Inebriated Drunk.

Inebriation Drunkenness.

Inebriety Habitual alcohol intoxication.

Infirm Drunk.

Influenced Drunk.

Inhale Allki To drink liquor.

Injay Gin.

Ink Cheap red wine.

Inked Drunk.

Inside Dope Liquor.

Insobriety *Same as* Inebriety.

Inspire To intoxicate.

Inspired Drunk.

Insult the Stomach Drink liquor.

Intemperance Drunkenness.

Intemperate Regular and excessive consumption of alcohol.

Into the Suds Drunk.

Intoxed *Same as* Intoxication.

Intoxication An altered state of consciousness caused by alcohol and resulting in a diminished capacity to function.

Inundated Drunk.

Invigorator Liquor.

Irish Cocktail Mickey Finn, drops of chloral hydrate surreptitiously dissolved in alcohol.

Irish coffee Coffee to which whiskey has been added.

Irish Earache Speech advocating abstinence from a reformed alcoholic.

Irish Toothache 1. Craving for alcohol. 2. A hangover.

Irish Whiskey Characteristic Irish liquor made by curing barley with charcoal and triple distilling.

Irish Wine Whiskey.

Irrigate To drink liquor.
Irrigate the Innards *Same as* Irrigate.
Irrigate, Will You Invitation to drink.
Irrigated Drunk.

J

Jack 1. Leather drinking mug. 2. Half or quarter-pint. 3. Liquor.

Jack Roll To rob one who is drunk.

Jack Roller, Jackroller Thief who robs drunks.

Jack Rouster, Jackrouster *Same as* Jack Roller.

Jackass Strong homemade liquor.

Jackass Brandy Potent homemade brandy.

Jacket, Jacket Can *Same as* Can.

Jag 1. Drunk. 2. An alcoholic. 3. Drinking spree. 4. Load of illicit liquor.

Jag, Have a Jag on 1. Drinking spree.

Jag Up To intoxicate.

Jagged, Jagged Up Drunk.

Jagster One on a drinking spree.

Jake 1. Drunkard. 2. Liquor.

Jake Hound Heavy drinker.

Jambled Drunk.

Jammed Drunk.

Jamboree Drinking spree party.

Jarred Drunk.

Jazz Up To add liquor to some other drink.

Jazzed, Jazzed Up Drunk.

Jellinek Formula Statistical procedure for estimating number of alcoholics in a community on the basis of incidence of deaths attributed to cirrhosis.

Jellinek's Disease Alcoholism. Named after E. M. Jellinek, a pioneer in alcohol research.

Jemmy John Jar for holding liquor.

Jenever Gin.

Jerk Beer To operate a liquor business.

Jerks Delirium Tremens.

Jeroboam Oversized wine bottle containing about four times the amount in a typical wine bottle.

Jerry Shop Abbreviation for Tom and Jerry shop.

Jersey Lightning 1. Applejack. 2. Potent liquor.

Jerusalem, Going to Drunk.

Jick Head, Jickhead An alcoholic.

Jig Juice Whiskey.

Jig Water Drink containing alcohol.

Jigger 1. Metal measuring cup (about 1 1/2 ounces used by bartenders in determing the amount to be used for a single drink. A jigger sometimes has two different sizes. The smaller size measures a "pony." 2. Drink of whiskey. 3. Secret still for making illicit liquor.

Jigger Boy Bartender.

Jiggered Drunk.

Jim Jams Delirium Tremens.

Jimmies Delirium Tremens.

Jimmy Illegal drinking place.

Jingle 1. Drinking binge. 2. To intoxicate.

Jingled Drunk.

Jinks Drinking spree or party.

Jinny Illicit liquor establishment.

Jitters Aftereffects of drinking.

Jocular Drunk.

John Alcoholic An alcoholic.

John Barleycorn Personification of whiskey made from barley.

John Hall Alcohol.

John W. Lumberman Drink of whiskey followed by beer.

Johnny Small glass of whiskey.

Joint Disreputable bar.

Joker Illicit liquor establishment.

Jolly Slightly drunk.

Jolly Nose An alcoholic.

Jolly Up To go on a drinking spree.

Jolt 1. Initial effect of alcohol. 2. Undiluted drink of liquor.

Joy Juice Liquor.

Joy Ride 1. Drinking spree. 2. Euphoric sensation from alcohol use.

Joy Rider One on a drinking spree.

Joy Water Liquor.

Jubilate To go on a drinking spree.

Jug Container for liquor.

Jug, On the Drinking excessively.

Jug Bitten Drunk.

Jug Goods Bottled whiskey sold in grocery stores.

Jug Juice Liquor.

Jug Up To drink intemperately.

Jugged Drunk.

Jugger An alcoholic.

Jug-steamed Drunk.

Juice Alcohol.

Juice Head An alcoholic.

Juice Joint A bar.

Juiced, Juiced Up Drunk.

Juicer Heavy drinker.

Juicy Drunk.

Julep Iced drink made by mixing various kinds of liquor and flavored with sugar and mint.

Jumbled Drunk.

Jump Bard To operate a liquor business.

Jumps Delirium Tremens.

Jungled Drunk.

Juniper Gin.

Juniper Juice Liquor, usually gin, which has the flavor of juniper berries.

Junk Liquor.

Junk Bottle Porter beer sold in a black-colored bottle.

K

K. T. Cocktail.

Kalmy, Kammy Wine or beer that has developed white particles on it while stored in a cask or bottle.

Katzenjammers Hangover.

Keep the Sails Up To remain sober.

Keep Your Nose Clean Don't drink alcohol.

Keg 1. Small cask for wine. 2. Container in which beer is held.

Keg Man Liquor magnate.

Keg Party 1. Party where there is a lot of drinking. 2. Party where beer is consumed.

Kennurd Drunk.

Kentucky Corn Corn whiskey.

Kentucky Fire Illicit whiskey.

Kentucky-fried Drunk.

Kerosene Liquor Moonshine whiskey contaminated with kerosene.

Kettle, Chase the Drunk.

Kettle, Hit his Drunk.

Key Up To add liquor to another beverage.

Keyed, Keyed Up Drunk.

Keyed to the Roof Drunk.

Kib'd Heels Drunk.

Kick 1. Strong drink of liquor. 2. Alcoholic content or reaction. 3. Chemical additives such as urea or nitrates in moonshine whiskey used to decrease fermentation time.

Kick in the Corn Alcoholic content or reaction.

Kick in the Gut Liquor.

Kick in the Wrist Drink of alcohol.

Kick up One's Heels To go on a drinking spree.

Kick Up the Devil Go on a drinking spree.

Kickapoo Joy Juice Illegally made whiskey.

Kicked in the Guts Drunk.

Kickless Non-alcoholic.

Kid Pocket flask of alcohol.

Kill To finish drinking whatever is left in a glass or bottle.

Kill a Fifth To drink a fifth gallon of liquor.

Kill a Marine To finish a bottle.

Kill a Shot To drink a glass of whiskey.

Kill One's Dog To get drunk.

Kill Priest Port wine.

Kill-devil Rum.

Killed Drunk.

King, Seen the French Drunk.

King, He's a Drunk.

King Alky Alcohol.

King is His Cousin Drunk.

King Kong Moonshine whiskey.

Kirschwasser Colorless brandy made from black cherries.

Kisky Drunk.

Kiss the Baby To drink liquor.

Kiss the Bottle To drink liquor

Kissed the Black Betty Drunk.

Kisserful Enough liquor to make one drunk.

Kitchen Illicit distillery.

Kitchen Boiler Homebrew.

Kited Drunk.

Knapt Drunk.

Knee-crawling drunk Very drunk.

Knee-walking drunk Very drunk.

Knitting Cup Cup of wine passed around during a wedding celebration.

Knock about the Bub To pass around the bottle.

Knock Down Strong beer or ale.

Knock Off To empty the glass or bottle.

Knock Out Drops Mixture of alcohol and chloral hydrate.

Knock Over a Drink To drink a glass of whiskey.

Knock-me-down Strong beer.

Knocked for a Loop Drunk.

Knocked off his Pins Drunk.

Knocked Out Drunk.

Knocked Over Drunk.

Knocked Up Drunk.

Knockered Drunk.

Knockout Drops Chloral hydrate added to alcohol.

Knows how the Cards are Dealt Heavy drinker.

Knows the Way Home Drunk.

Korsakoff's Psychosis Mental disturbance involving loss of memory and initiative resulting from chronic and excessive alcohol consumption.

Korsakoff's Syndrome *Same as* Korsakoff's Psychosis.

Kummel Liqueur made from grain and flavored with caraway and cummin.

L

L. L. Whiskey Very good whiskey.

Label Faker One who counterfeits liquor labels.

Lace To add liquor to another beverage like coffee or tea.

Lace-curtain drinker One who does most of his drinking in a cocktail lounge.

Laced 1. Alcohol added to another beverage. 2. Drunk.

Lady Dacre's Wine Gin.

Lady May Gallon of whiskey.

Lager Type of aged beer introduced by the Germans.

Laid Out Drunk.

Laid Right Out Drunk.

Laid to the Bone Drunk.

Lambrusco Sweet red wine from Italy.

Lamb's Wool Hot drink popular in England and the colonies in 1600s–1700s; made with wine, spices, sugar, and roasted apples floating on the surface, served in a large bowl. Sometimes ale was substituted for wine. Also known as Yard of Flannel.

Lame Drunk.

Lamp Oil Whiskey.

Lap 1. Any alcohol beverage. 2. Gin. 3. To drink heavily.

Lap Dog Heavy drinker.

Lap in the Gutter Drunk.

Lap It Up To drink intemperately.

Lap the Gutter 1. To drink too much alcohol. 2. To become drunk to the point where one cannot stand.

Lapper An alcoholic.

Lappy Drunk.

Lappy Cull An alcoholic.

Large Head An alcoholic.

Lark Drinking spree.

Lathered Drunk.

Laughing Jag Given to laughter while under the influence of alcohol.

Laughing Soup Liquor.

Laughing Water Champagne.

Law, the Agent of the Federal Treasury Department's Alcohol Tax unit.

Lay the Dust To drink alcohol.

Leaner Destitute alcoholic who does not have money for even the poorest accommodations.

Leaning Drunk.

Leaping, Leaping Up Drunk.

Lear Beer Prohibitionist.

Leary Drunk.

Leery Drunk.

Lees Sediment formed at the bottom of a wine barrel or bottle after fermentation.

Legger Bootlegger.

Leggery Illegal drinking place.

Leggs, Makes Indentures with his Drunk.

Legless Drunk.

Leist Drink liquor.

Less Noise, Less Noise! Toast.

Lest We Forget Toast.

Let 'er Go To go on a drinking spree.

Let 'er Go Gallagher To go on a drinking spree.

Let 'er Snort To go on a drinking spree.

Let 'er Tear To go on a drinking spree.

Let Go To go on a drinking spree.

Let Off Steam To go on a drinking spree.

Let Us Drive Another Nail Invitation to drink.

Let Us Get There Invitation to drink.

Let Us Have One Invitation to drink.

Let Us Irrigate Invitation to drink.

Let Us See a Man About a Dog Invitation to drink.

Let Us Stimulate Invitation to drink.

Leth Bringer Alcohol.

Level Off To drink to a point of desired intoxication and no more.

Leveled Drunk.

Lickspigot Ale-house keeper.

Lie in the Gutter To get very drunk.

Liebfraumilch Inexpensive German table wine.

Life Preserver Pocket flask of liquor.

Lift 1. Drink taken as a stimulant. 2. Alcoholic content or reaction.

Lifted Drunk.

Light Drunk.

Light Beer Beer containing less than the usual amount of alcohol.

Light-Bodied Whiskey with a low congener content.

Light-headed Drunk.

Light Wet Gin.

Light Whiskey Whiskey that lacks the flavoring of traditional whiskey.

Lightning 1. Potent alcoholic beverage. 2. Cheap whiskey.

Lightning Flash Cheap whiskey.

Lightning Lush Strong liquor.

Likker Liquor.

Likker Factory Bar.

Likker Pug Liquor abstainer.

Likkered, Likkered-up Drunk.

Likkerous Drunk.

Likker-soaked Drunk.

Likkerteer Liquor racketeer.

Likker-up Drunkenness.

Likkerish Tooth Desire for liquor.

Limber Drunk.

Lime To clean the inside of fermenters.

Limp Drunk.

Lined Drunk.

Lion Drunk Drunk and quarrelsome.

Liqueur Sweet alcoholic beverage containing between 20 to 60% alcohol, usually consumed as an after dinner drink. Made by mixing or distilling alcohol with fruits, juices, flowers, plants, etc.

Liquid Courage Liquor.

Liquid Fire Liquor.

Liquid Fuel Liquor.

Liquid Joy Liquor.

Liquified Drunk.

Liquor 1. Distilled alcohol. 2. To take a drink. 3. Alcoholic beverages which have been made by distillation.

Liquor, In Drunk.

Liquor Head Alcoholic.

Liquor One's Boots To drink alcohol before a journey.

Liquor Plug Heavy drinker.

Liquor Store Store in which various kinds of alcohol are sold.

Liquor Struck Drunk.

Liquor Up To get drunk.

Liquored, Liquored Up Drunk.

Liquorification Drunkenness.

Liquorish Drunk.

Liquorium An elaborate bar.

Listing Drunk.

Lit Drunk.

Lit a Bit Drunk.

Lit to the Gills Drunk.

Lit to the Guards Drunk.

Lit to the Gunnels Drunk.

Lit Up Drunk.

Lit up like a Cathedral Drunk.

Lit up like a Christmas Tree Drunk.

Lit up like a Church Drunk.

Lit up like a High Mass Drunk.

Lit up like a Kite Drunk.

Lit up like a Skyscraper Drunk.

Lit up like a Store Window Drunk.

Lit up like Broadway Drunk.

Lit up like Main Street Drunk.

Lit up like the Catholic Church Drunk.

Lit up like the Sky Drunk.

Lit up like Times Square Drunk.

Little Brown Jug Bottle of liquor.

Little Church Around the Corner Local bar.

Little Tight Slightly drunk.

Little Whack Small drink of liquor.

Little Woozy Slightly drunk.

Live Marine Bottle of liquor.

Live Well, to Drunk.

Livener Drink taken as a stimulant.

Load of Pig Iron Shipment of illegally made liquor.

Load One's Card To get drunk.

Load under the Skin Enough liquor to make one drunk.

Loaded Drunk.

Loaded for Bear Drunk.

Loaded his Cart Drunk.

Loaded to the Barrel Drunk.

Loaded to the Earlobes Drunk.

Loaded to the Gills Drunk.

Loaded to the Guards Drunk.

Loaded to the Gunnels Drunk.

Loaded to the Gunwales Drunk.

Loaded to the Hat Drunk.

Loaded to the Muzzle Drunk.

Loaded to the Plimsoll Mark Drunk.

Local Option Community's prerogative to decide whether sale of alcohol within its jurisdiction will be permitted.

Lock-legged Drunk.

Log and Copper Whiskey Whiskey made by heating whiskey mash above logs placed under a copper pipe.

Logged Drunk.

Lone Eagle Solitary drinker.

Lonesome Private or surreptitious drinker.

Long Drag Large glass or drink of liquor.

Long Neck Whiskey or rum bottle.

Long Necker Bottle of alcohol.

Long One Large drink of liquor.

Long Pull *Same as* Long One.

Long Sleever *Same as* Long One.

Long Stale Drunk Extended drinking binge.

Look Blue About the Gills Drunk.

Look Down the Neck of a Bottle To drink whiskey straight from the bottle.

Look through Rose-Colored Glasses To drink liquor.

Looking Glass Drinking Drinking at the bar.

Lookout *Same as* Guard.

Loony Drunk.

Loop Drinking spree.

Looped Drunk.

Looped-legged Drunk.

Loop-legged Drunk.

Loopy Drunk.

Loose 1. On a drinking spree. 2. Relaxed by alcohol.

Loose in the Hilt Drunk.

Loppy Drunk.

Lord, Drunk as a Very drunk.

Lordly Drunk.

Lost Cause 18th Amendment.

Lost his Rudder Drunk.

Lost Memory Cheap wine.

Lotion Alcohol.

Lousy Drunk Very drunk.

Love Pot Drunkard.

Loveage Leftover remains in glasses poured down holes in a bar.

Love-Dovey Amorously drunk.

Low Bottom Drunk Alcoholic who has no self-respect and has reached the lowest level of degradation.

Low Country Soldier Heavy drinker.

Low Talk Illegal bar.

Low Wines Early part of the distillation process. Contains a low alcohol content.

Lower Liquor To drink liquor.

Lubricate To drink alcohol.

Lubricated Drunk.

Lubricating Room Room maintained by liquor lobby near legislatures in various states where elected officials were given free drinks and lobbied to vote against prohibition measures.

Lumped Drunk.

Lumpy Drunk.

Lush 1. Drunkenness. 2. A drunkard.

Lush Crib A bar.

Lush Diver Robber of intoxicated persons.

Lush Hound Habitual drinker.

Lush House A bar.

Lush Job To rob one who is intoxicated.

Lush Roller Thief who robs drunks.

Lush Toucher *Same as* Lush Roller.

Lush Up Intoxicate.

Lush Worker *Same as* Lush Roller.

Lushed, Lushed Up Drunk.

Lusher An alcoholic.

Lushey, Lushie, Lushy 1. An alcoholic. 2. Drunk.

Lushing Cove A drunkard.

Lushing Man Heavy drinker.

Lushington A drunkard.

Lushy Drunk.

M

M.A. Morning after, referring to hangover.

Maceration Process of making liqueur by steeping fruit in alcohol.

Mad Greek One who drank often and considerably.

Madam Geneva Gin.

Madam Gin Gin.

MADD Mothers Against Drunk Driving.

Madeira Fortified dessert wine from Madeira island. Aged in heated warehouses for six months.

Madeirized A mature wine that has turned tawny due to aging and smells somewhat like Madeira wine.

Magnum Large wine bottle about twice the size of an ordinary bottle.

Mail Runner *See* Running the Mail.

Mainbrace is Well-Spliced Drunk.

Maine Law First statewide prohibition law in U.S. Passed in 1851.

Main-sheet Brandy.

Make a Jug To get enough money, usually by panhandling, to buy wine or whiskey.

Make a Night of It To go on an all-night drinking spree.

Make a Run To go to the liquor store for a bottle.

Make a Strike Rob someone who is drunk.

Make Hell Pop Loose To go on a drinking spree.

Make Hey-Hey To go on a drinking spree.

Make It a Creep To order a glass of draft beer.

Make Shift Liquor.

Make Things Look Crimson To go on a drinking spree.

Make's One See Double and Feel Single Strong liquor.

Making M's and T's Reeling drunk.

Making Scallops Reeling drunk.

Malaga Dessert wine from Malaga, Spain.

Malmsey Type of Madeira wine.

Malt 1. Beer. 2. Barley that has germinated. First stage in making beer. 3. To drink beer.

Malt beverage Beverage made from malt that has not fermented.

Malt House 1. Place where malt is brewed. 2. Tavern.

Malt Is above Wheat with Him Slightly drunk.

Malt liquor Alcoholic beverage made from malt with a higher alcohol and sweeter taste content than beer.

Malted Drunk on beer.

Maltician Distiller.

Maltimillionaire Wealthy brewer.

Maltster One who makes malt.

Maltworm Drunkard.

Malty Drunk on beer.

Mamie Taylor Liquor.

Mandarine Liqueur made from tangerines.

Man-Sized Order Large glass or drink of liquor.

Marine Bottle of beer or liquor.

Marine Soldier Full liquor bottle.

Marsala Dessert wine from Italy.

Marshal Agent of the Federal Treasury department.

Martin Drunk Very drunk.

Martini Mixed drink made with gin, vermouth, and bitters.

Martini Alcoholic An alcoholic who has high social status.

Mash Grain material to which water has been added in making liquor or beer.

Mash Back *Same as* Double Back.

Mashing 1. Making moonshine whiskey. 2. Mixing corn grain with rye and limestone water and then scalding the mixture with fresh hot material from a prior distillation.

Mashing Tub, Mashing Tun Tub in which mash is placed so that starches and proteins will be broken down prior to brewing.

MAST See Michigan Alcoholism Screening Test.

Materials Whiskey punch.

Mature Wine that has been aged to bring out its best qualities.

Maudlin Drunk and crying.

Mauled Very drunk.

Max 1. Gin. 2. Potent liquor.

Mazer Drinking cup made of maple wood.

Mead Wine made from honey.

Mealer One who drinks alcoholic beverages only during meals.

Medicine Alcohol.

Medium Dryish Favoring Prohibition.

Meitei-sho Drunkenness without alcohol consumption. Caused by a normal intestinal yeast, *Candida albicans*, that is very high in a small minority of individuals and causes intestinal carbohydrates to be transformed into alcohol.

Melancholism Blend of melancholy and alcoholism.

Mellow 1. Relaxed feeling produced by alcohol. 2. Drunk.

Mellowness Drunkenness.

Melted Very drunk.

Merchandise Liquor.

Mercurey Red wine from France.

Meridian Noon drink, usually punch.

Merry Drunk.

Merry as a Grigg Drunk.

Merry Comrade Drinking companion.

Merry Hell To go on a drinking spree.

Merry Pin, On a Drunk.

Merry-Go-Round Drinking spree.

Merrymake To go on a drinking spree.

Metabolism Biochemical process by which alcohol is broken down. First breakdown product or metabolite of alcohol is acetaldehyde.

Methanol *See* Wood Alcohol.

Metheglin Spiced honey wine.

Methodist Hellenium Prohibition era.

Methodistconated Drunk.

Methuselah Large wine bottle with the capacity of eight normal wine bottles.

Michael Hip flask for whiskey.

Michael Finn Strong drink of liquor.

Michigan Alcoholism Screening Test (MAST) Question and answer test for deciding if someone is an alcoholic.

Mick To give someone a Mickey Finn.

Mickey Small bottle or flask for liquor.

Mickey Finn Alcoholic drink to which chloral hydrate has been added.

Mickey Flynn *Same as* Mickey Finn.

Middle Liquors Most desirable portion of the distillation process; the part that is not discarded.

Middling Drunk.

Middlings Livestock feed used as substitute for grain when grain is unavailable for distillation.

Milled Drunk.

Minnehaha Alcohol.

Mippitate Drink Liquor.

Misery Gin.

Mission Rehabilitation center for homeless men, many of whom are alcoholics.

Mix Mixed or adulterated drink.

Mixed Drinks Alcoholic beverages, usually wine or liquor, to which other substances are added.

Mixed Up Mixed or adulterated drink.

Mixer Bartender.

Mixologist Someone adept at preparing alcoholic drinks.

Mizzled Drunk.

Moaning After Morning after a drinking spree.

Mobbi A drink made from potatoes.

Mocus Drunk.

Modest Quencher Drink made with whiskey and water.

Moist Anti-prohibitionist.

Moist Around the Edges Drunk.

Moist 'Un Drunk.

Moisten the Clay To drink liquor.

Moisterous Antiprohibition.

Moisture Liquor.

Mokus Liquor.

Monday Blues Aftereffects of a Sunday night carousal.

Mongrel Mixture Cocktail.

Monkey Cask containing rum.

Monkey Juice Cheap wine.

Monkey Pump Straw used in sucking liquor from a cask or bottle.

Monkey Swill Liquor.

Monuments, Raised his Drunk.

Moon Moonshine.

Mooney 1. Whiskey. 2. Dreamy from liquor. 3. Drunk.

Moon-eyed Drunk.

Moonlight Illicit liquor.

Moonlight Inn Place where alcohol is sold illegally.

Moonlighter Bootlegger.

Moons, Seen a Flock of Drunk.

Moonshine 1. Alcohol product on which no taxes have been paid. 2. Whiskey, usually cheap, containing a high alcohol content and produced at home. Usually used in reference to whiskey made from corn or rye, or brandy made from apples or peaches.

Moonshine Joint Place where liquor is sold illegally.

Moonshiner Maker or seller of illicit whiskey.

Moonshiner's Gopher Someone who sells illegal liquor.

Moose Milk Moonshine.

Mop 1. A drinking party. 2. A drunkard. 3. A prolonged period of drunkenness.

Mop Up To drink.

Moppy Drunk.

Mops and Brooms Drunk.

Morning Bitters Popular eighteenth century drink in southern U.S. made with rum, brandy, whiskey, and bitter bark of trees. Consumed on a regular basis as an alcohol beverage and to ward off malaria.

Morning Rouser *Same as* Eye-opener.

Morning's Morning *Same as* Eye-opener.

Mother Wine or beer that has developed a thickish scum on its surface while stored in a cask or bottle.

Mother's Milk Gin.

Mothers Against Drunk Driving (MADD) Community action group organized to change laws against drunk driving.

Motorman's Glove High-proof whiskey.

Mountain Malaga wine.

Mountain Dew 1. Moonshine. 2. Potent liquor.

Mountain Teapot Small moonshine still.

Mouth, Have a To feel the effect of drinking.

Mouthwash Liquor.

Mr. Haig Straight scotch whiskey.

M.T. Empty liquor bottle.

Muck To get drunk.

Muddled Drunk.

Muddler Drunkard.

Muddy Drunk.

Mug Blot Drunkard.

Mug House A tavern.

Mugg Blotts Drunk.

Mugged Drunk.

Muggy Drunk.

Mug's Game Alcoholism.

Mule 1. Whiskey made from corn. 2. Marihuana mixed with whiskey.

Mule and Aqua Cheap liquor.

Mull To warm and sweeten wine.

Mulled 1. Heated wine drinks. 2. Drunk.

Mulled Up Drunk.

Mum Strong ale made from wheat malt.

Mumbo Popular drink in early America made with rum, water, and lumps of sugar.

Murky Drunk.

Muscatel A sweet wine from Spain.

Muskabooby Muscatel wine.

Muskadoo, Muskadoodle Muscatel wine.

Musky, Musky Pete Muscatel wine.

Must Grape juice that has not completely fermented.

Mustika Potent liquor.

Musty Moldy, unpleasant smell in wines.

Muzzler Liquor.

Muzzy Drunk.

N

Nail, Off the Drunk.

Nail in the Coffin A drink.

Naked Undiluted Liquor.

Name It Invitation to drink.

Name Yours Invitation to drink.

Nanny Goat Sweat Liquor.

Nantz Brandy.

Napoleon Brandy Brandy that has aged many years.

Nappy, Noppy 1. Drunk. 2. Strong ale. 3. Inebriating.

Nase Drunk.

National Association of State Alcohol and Drug Abuse Directors (NASADAD) Association to promote exchange of information and a united front in attempts to influence federal narcotics and alcohol policy.

National Institute of Mental Health (NIMH) U.S. Federal agency responsible for promoting mental health, prevention and treatment of mental illness, and rehabilitation of the mentally ill.

National Institute on Alcohol Abuse and Alcoholism (NIAAA) U.S. agency responsible for prevention, control, and treatment of alcohol abuse and rehabilitation of alcohol abusers.

Naturalized Alky Denatured alcohol.

Nazie Drunk.

Nazie Mort Drunken woman.

Nazy Drunk.

Nazy Cove An alcoholic.

Nazy Nob A drunkard.

Near Beer Beer with 0.5 percent alcohol content or less.

Neat Unadulterated.

Nebuchadnezzar Very large wine bottle equal in capacity to twenty ordinary bottles.

Neck Oil 1. Beer. 2. Whiskey.

Nectar Liquor.

Nectar of the Gods Liquor.

Needle 1. To add alcohol to some other drink. 2. Beer to which alcohol has been added.

Needle Beer Beer to which alcohol has been added.

Needle Joint Liquor establishment which needles beer.

Needle Man One who needles beer.

Needling Simulating the aging of whiskey by passing an electric current through a needle placed in the barrel of liquor.

Negus English drink popular in 1800s made with boiling water, wine (usually port), sugar, lemon juice, and spices.

Nelson's Blood Rum.

Neutral spirits Distillate made from redistilled whiskey, brandy, or rum. Contains 190 proof or more alcohol and does not have any distinctive taste, color, or smell. Used to blend with other alcohol beverages to increase their alcohol content.

Never Fear Beer.

Newer Freedom Repeal.

Next Morning Suisses Hangover.

Nig Gin.

Nigger Gin Liquor with high alcohol content.

Nightcap A drink taken just before going to bed.

Night Mare, Got the Drunk.

Nimptopsical Drunk.

Nimtopsical Drunk.

Ninety-nine.nine (99.9) Add liquor to a nonalcoholic drink.

Nip Small drink.

Nip at the Cable Drink taken in secret aboard ship.

Nipped Drunk.

Nipper One who takes small drinks throughout the day.

Nipper-kin A glass for drinking alcohol beverages.

Nippitate Strong ale or liquor.

Nippitatum, Nippitato *Same as* Nippitate.

Niptopsical Drunk.

No Daylight Full glass of beer.

No Heeltaps To finish a drink of liquor.

Noble 1. High quality. 2. Mature wine.

Noble Experiment 18th Amendment.

Nockum Stiff Bourbon.

Noddy-headed Drunk.

Nog Any mixed drink containing egg.

Noggin A drink.

Nominate your Pizen Invitation to drink.

Non Compos Drunk.

Nose is Dirty Drunk.

Nose Paint Liquor.

Nose Paint Factory Liquor establishment.

Nose Painting Drinking liquor.

Not All There Drunk.

Not Heel Over To remain sober.

Not Show One's Drinks Not easily overcome by liquor.

Not Suffering Drunk.

Numb Drunk.

Nursemaid Alcoholism counselor.

Nut, On the On skid row.

Nuts Drunk.

Nutty Drunk.

N.Y.D. Not Yet Diagnosed. Term used to avoid diagnosis of alcoholism.

Nystagmus Involuntary rapid eye movement commonly associated with excessive drinking.

O

Oak Char Charring of inside of oak barrels before using them for storing bourbon. Charring imparts flavor to the whiskey.

Oasis A bar.

Obarni Scalded honey wine.

Obfuscated Drunk.

Obfusticated Drunk.

Oddish Drunk.

Oenologist One who studies wine.

Oenology Study of wine.

Oenomania Craving for wine.

Oenometer Instrument for measuring amount of alcohol in wine.

Oenophilist Alcoholic who primarily drinks wine.

Oenophobist One who has a fear of drinking wine.

Off Drunk.

Off a Drunk Time after a drinking spree.

Off a Hummer *Same as* Off a Drunk.

Off at the Nail Drunk.

Off his Bean Drunk.

Off his Feet Drunk.

Off it Abstaining from alcohol.

Off the Bottle To abstain from liquor.

Off the Deep End Drunk.

Off the Wagon Drinking alcohol after an extended period of abstinence.

Off to the Races Drunk.

Offall Weak beer.

Oh-be-joyful Liquor.

Oh-be-rich-an'-happy Liquor.

Oh My Near Beer.

Oil Make drunk.

Oil Head An alcoholic.

Oil of Barley Beer.

Oil of Joy Liquor.

Oil the Clay To drink liquor.

Oil the Goozle To drink liquor.

Oil the Lapper To drink liquor.

Oil the Swallow To drink liquor.

Oil the Tonsils To drink liquor.

Oil the Whistle To drink liquor.

Oiled Drunk.

Oiler Drunkard.

Oinomania Craving for alcohol.

Old Crow 1. A drink. 2. Brand name for bourbon.

Old Metheglin Dark-brown wine made from honey.

Old Peach Liquor made from peaches.

Old Sneak Inexpensive fortified wine.

Old Soak Older alcoholic.

Old Tom Gin.

Old whiskey Whiskey that has aged.

On Slightly drunk.

On a Bat Drinking a large amount of alcohol in a short amount of time; a drinking spree.

On a Bender On a drinking spree.

On a Binge On a drinking spree.

On a Brannigan On a drinking spree.

On a Bum On a drinking spree.

On a Bus On a drinking spree.

On a Bust On a drinking spree.

On a Drunk On a drinking spree.

On a Jag On a drinking spree.

On a Racket On a drinking spree.

On a Skate On a drinking spree.

On a Spree On a drinking spree.

On a Tear On a drinking spree.

On a Tipple On a drinking spree.

On a Toot On a drinking spree.

On a Weeping Jag On a drinking spree.

On his Ass Drunk.

On his Ear Drunk.

On his Fourth Drunk.

On his Last Legs Drunk.

On his Way Out Drunk.

On the Beer On a beer drinking spree.

On the Blink Drunk.

On the Booze Drinking heavily and often.

On the Choo-Choo Abstaining from liquor.

On the Floor Drunk.

On the Grog *Same as* On the Booze.

On the Juice *Same as* On the Booze.

On the Lee Lurch Drunk.

On the Loose On a drinking spree.

On the Rampage State of uproarious intoxication.

On the Rocks Liquor poured over ice cubes.

On the Sauce 1. On a drinking spree. 2. *Same as* On the Booze.

On the Shikker Drunk.

On the Wagon Abstaining from drinking.

One across the Board Drink served at a bar.

One Down 1. Glass of draught beer. 2. Straight rye.

One-eared Wine that is not aged enough.

One for the Road One more drink (usually after having had several) before going home.

One on the House A drink at the house's expense.

One on the Merry-go-round One who is on a drinking spree.

One Out of the Barrel Strong drink of liquor.

One-over-eight Drunk.

One Straight From the Shoulder Strong drink of liquor.

One Too Many Drunk.

One Up Large glass of beer ready to be served.

Onion, Smelt of an Drunk.

Oof Alcoholic content or reaction.

Optimistically Dry Favoring Prohibition.

Order of Good Templars First international temperance organization started in 1851 in Utica, New York.

Ordinaire Common wine of France.

Organic disorder Impaired function due to known pathological condition.

Organize To make drunk.

Organized Drunk.

Orie-eyed Drunk.

Ork-Orks 1. Hangover. 2. Delirium Tremens.

Oscillated Drunk.

Ossified Drunk.

Ostler ale Weak ale.

Out 1. Slightly drunk. 2. Glass in which whiskey is served.

Out Cold Comatose from drinking.

Out for the Count *Same as* Out Cold.

Out Like a Lamp Drunk.

Out Like a Light *Same as* Out Like a Lamp.

Out of his Element Drunk.

Out of his Mind Drunk.

Out of it Drunk.

Out of One's Mind Drunk.

Out of the Barrel Undiluted whiskey.

Out of the Picture Drunk.

Out of the Way Drunk.

Out on the Roof Drunk.

Out to Lunch Drunk.

Outage Material which evaporates from a barrel during the aging process.

Outfit *Same as* Still.

Outpatient Patient living in the outside community while receiving treatment.

Ouzo Anise-flavored liqueur from Greece.

Over the Bay Drunk.

Over the Mark Drunk.

Overboard Drunk.

Overcome Drunk.

Overdone Drunk.

Overloaded Drunk.

Overseas Drunk.

Overseen Drunk.

Overserved Drunk.

Overset Drunk.

Overshot Drunk.

Overtake To make drunk.

Overtaken Drunk.

Overwined Drunk.

Owl, Drunk as an Drunk.

Owled Drunk.

Owl-eyed Drunk.

Oxycrocium Drunk.

P

Pack Rum.

Pack a (mean) Wallop 1. Contain alcohol. 2. To make a strong drink.

Package, Have a Package on Drunk.

Package Store Store in which alcoholic beverages are sold in bottles or cans for consumption elsewhere, and often packaged in plain brown bags.

Packaged Drunk.

Pain Killer Liquor.

Paint To drink.

Paint his Nose To drink whiskey intemperately.

Paint his Tonsils To drink whiskey.

Paint Remover Strong liquor.

Paint the Town To celebrate boisterously by drinking a lot of alcohol.

Paint the Town Red *Same as* Paint the Town.

Palatic Drunk.

Pale Near-beer.

Palled Very drunk.

Panhandle To beg for money to be spent on liquor.

Panther Gin.

Panther Piss Cheap whiskey.

Panther Sweat *Same as* Panther Piss.

Panther's Breath *Same as* Moonshine.

Pantry Drinker One who drinks alcohol alone.

Paraldy Paraldehyde, drug used to treat withdrawal from alcohol.

Paralytic Very drunk.

Paralyzed *Same as* Paralyzed.

Paralyzer Strong liquor.

Paranoia Condition characterized by extreme suspiciousness of being watched and fear of being arrested.

Parboiled Drunk.

Parliament Whiskey Illicit whiskey.

Party Gathering of two or more people to drink together.

Partying Any planned gathering in which consumption of alcohol is a main reason for congregating.

Pass Brandy Brandy made in Texas.

Pass Out Get dead drunk.

Pass Out of the Picture Get very drunk.

Pass the Bottle To drink liquor.

Pass Whiskey Whiskey made in Texas.

Passed out Comatose from drinking too much.

Past Gone Drunk.

Pasted Drunk.

Pasteurization Heating beer or wine to stop further fermentation.

Pathological intoxication Unusual reaction to alcohol in which individual may become intoxicated after drinking very little.

Paunch, Wasted his Drunk.

Pay the Freight To pay for one's own drinks.

Peckish Drunk.

Peddler Liquor dealer.

Pee-eyed Drunk.

Peekish Drunk.

Peg 1. A drink. 2. Mixture of brandy and soda water. 3. To drink to excess.

Peg Lower, Go a To have another drink.

Pegger A drunkard.

Peonied Drunk.

Pep Drink of whiskey or brandy.

Pep Up To drink liquor.

Pepless Nonalcoholic.

Pepped Drunk.

Pepped Up Liquor added to another drink.

Pepper Upper Drink taken as a stimulant.

Peppy Potent.

Pepst Drunk.

Performer Someone who becomes unruly after drinking alcohol.

Periodic alcoholism Uncontrollable craving for alcohol during specific periods with periods of abstinence or moderate drinking in between.

Perked Drunk.

Perkin Beer.

Pernod Anise-flavored aperitif produced as a substitute for absinthe.

Perry Fermented pear juice.

Pete *Same as* Sneaky Pete.

Petrificated Drunk.

Petrified Drunk.

Petty Warrant Beer Beer obtained when English seamen docked at foreign ports.

Pharaoh, Contending with Drunk.

Pharmacokinetics Study of the absorption, distribution, metabolism, and elimination of substances such as alcohol from the body.

Pharo Potent alcohol beverage.

Philippians, Been among the Drunk.

Philistines, Been among the Drunk.

Phlegm Cutter Potent alcoholic beverage.

Phlegm Disperser *Same as* Phlegm Cutter.

Physic Alcoholic drink.

Pick-Me-Up Drink taken as a stimulant.

Pick-Up *Same as* Pick-Me-Up.

Pickle Drunkenness.

Pickle Oneself To get dead drunk.

Pickled Drunk.

Pickling Simulating aging by placing oak chips or charcoal into moonshine whiskey to give it color and flavor.

Pidgeon-eyed Drunk.

Pied Drunk.

Pie-eyed Drunk.

Piffed Drunk.

Pifficated Drunk.

Piffled Drunk.

Pifflicated *Same as* Piffled.

Pig Illicit bar.

Pigeon New member of Alcoholics Anonymous assigned to another member with more experience.

Pigeon-eyed Drunk.

Piggy-back Doubling Distilling moonshine more than once.

Pilfered Drunk.

Pillman One who combines barbiturates with alcohol.

Pillow-cup *Same as* Nightcap.

Piment Wine drink made with honey and spices.

Pin, to To drink one's share.

Pin Drunk Drunk.

Pine Top Cheap whiskey.

Pink Wine Champagne.

Pinked Drunk.

Pinko Drunk.

Pint Peddler Bootlegger.

Pious Drunk.

Pipe Large wine cask with tapered ends.

Piped Drunk.

Pipped Drunk.

Pirate Liquor runner on the high seas.

Piss Inferior liquor.

Piss Factory A bar.

Piss Maker Liquor.

Pissed Drunk.

Pissed to the Eyes *Same as* Pissed.

Pixilated Drunk.

Pizen Whiskey.

Plain Undiluted whiskey.

Plain Drunk Drunk.

Plant Place where liquor was stored.

Plaster To intoxicate.

Plastered Drunk.

Plated Drunk.

Play the Greek Drink to excess.

Played Out Drunk.

Playing the Sovereign Giving out free drinks for political favors.

Pleasantly Jingled Drunk.

Pledge 1. Toast. 2. Vow of abstinence from alcohol.

Plonk Cheap wine.

Plonked Drunk.

Plotzed Drunk.

Ploughed Drunk.

Ploughed Under Drunk.

Plowed Drunk.

Ploxed Drunk.

Pluck Wine.

Pocket Pistol Flask of liquor.

Pogie, Pogy Drunk.

Poggled Drunk.

Poison Inferior liquor.

Poison Up To drink liquor.

Pole, Up the Drunk.

Policeman Antabuse.

Polished Drunk.

Polite Drunk.

Pollute To make drunk.

Polluted Drunk.

Ponge Beer.

Pongelo Beer.

Pony 1. Small glass of liquor. 2. Measuring glass for dispensing liquor.

Poop Out To get dead drunk.

Poor Boy Small glass of whiskey.

Pop-eyed Drunk.

Pop Highball Combination of alcohol and soda.

Pop Wallah Abstainer.

Pop Wine Sweet, fruit-tasting wine.

Popskull 1. Illicitly produced whiskey, usually made in private homes during Prohibition era. 2. Whiskey.

Port Fortified sweet wine.

Porter Dark-brown bitter ale similar to, but more carbonated than, stout.

Posset Drink made with hot wine or beer and hot milk to which various spices and sugar were added.

Pot 1. Container for drink, abbreviation for pottle. 2. A drink. 3. Abbreviation for pot still.

Pot Companion Fellow drinker.

Pot Shaken Drunk.

Pot Still 1. Still made of copper kettle, coil, and water jacket. 2. Still using direct heat from fire rather than steam.

Pot Valiant *Same as* Dutch courage.

Pot Walloper Drunkard.

Potboy Waiter in a bar.

Poteen Irish whiskey.

Potency Strength of action. The quantity of alcoholic beverage producing a particular response. The smaller the amount of substance, the greater the potency.

Potent Stuff Liquor.

Potentiation Combined effect of two or more drugs that produces a greater effect than either alone.

Potfury Drunkenness.

Pot-hardy Drunk.

Potheen Illicit whiskey.

Pothouse Disreputable bar.

Potkinight One who becomes belligerent when drunk.

Potleech Drunkard.

Potman Drunkard.

Potomania Craving for alcohol.

Pots, Among the Drunk.

Pots, In the Drunk.

Pots On Drunk.

Potshot Drunk.

Potsick Drunk.

Potsville Drunk.

Potted Drunk.

Pottle Container for ale or beer holding about two quarts.

Potty Drunk.

Potulent Drunk.

Potvaliant *Same as* Dutch Courage.

Pot-verdugo Drunkenness.

Pour-Out Man Bartender.

Pour Up To pour moonshine into containers for sale.

Powder Drink containing alcohol.

Powder Up To get drunk.

Powdered Drunk.

Powie Alcoholic content or reaction.

Prairie Dew Whiskey.

Prairie Schooner Large mug of beer.

Preacher's Lye Potent moonshine whiskey.

Pre-Prohi Bottled in bond liquor.

Prescription Whiskey Liquor obtained by prescription during Prohibition.

Preserve To intoxicate.

Preserved Drunk.

Pre-stoned Drunk.

Pretty Drunk Drunk.

Pretty Far Gone Drunk.

Pretty Happy Drunk.

Pretty High Drunk.

Pretty Well-plowed Drunk.

Pretty Well-primed Drunk.

Pre-Volstead Before Prohibition.

Pre-war Stuff Liquor manufactured prior to World War I.

Price Cost of a drink.

Priddy Drunk.

Prime To offer alcohol to remove inhibitions and to accomplish sexual seduction.

Prime-Up To drink liquor intemperately.

Prime Yourself Invitation to take a drink.

Primed Drunk.

Primed to the Barrel Drunk.

Primed to the Muzzle Drunk.

Primed to the Trigger Drunk.

Primitive Undiluted whiskey.

Problem drinker 1. One whose drinking results in family difficulty, job-related problems, or health-related problems. 2. An alcoholic.

Prohi Agent of the Federal Treasury Department.

Prohibishop Bishop who favored Prohibition.

Prohibition 1. Banning by statutory or constitutional law of saloons and/or of liquor trade. 2. Attitude favoring legal coercion on moral grounds.

Prohibition Amendment Eighteenth amendment to U.S. constitution outlawing manufacture, distribution, and sale of alcohol.

Prohibition Error Prohibition Era.

Prohibitionist Individual in favor of prohibition.

Pro-Inhibition Blend of prohibition and inhibition.

Proof Measure of the amount of alcohol in a solution, twice the alcohol concentration.

Proof gallon Gallon of potable solution containing standard U.S. measure (100 proof) on which Federal excise taxes are collected.

Propination Toast.

Prosit Toast.

Prosperity, In his Drunk.

Prowl, On the Searching for money to buy drinks.

Prune Juice Potent alcoholic beverage.

Pruned Drunk.

Pruno Fermented prune juice.

Psychoactive Any chemical agent that acts on the mind.

Psychopharmacology Branch of pharmacology concerned with substances that affect behavior or subjective experience.

Psychosis Severe mental disturbance in which individual loses touch with reality and may experience hallucinations or delusions.

Pub Commonly used term in England for a local tavern or bar. Public house.

Pub Crawl Visiting all the bars in a town.

Public Drunkenness Intoxication in public.

Public House *See* Pub.

Publican Owner of a pub.

Pudding Bag, Eat a Drunk.

Puggy Drunk.

Puke Material that sometimes boils over from the still into the connections.

Pull A drink.

Pull a Daniel Boone To get drunk.

Pull a Shut-eye To get drunk.

Pull Out Dismantling a still to avoid detection.

Pull the Still *Same as* Pull Out.

Puller Liquor smuggler.

Pummie Moonshine brandy made from fermented fruit or fruit juice.

Punch Mixture of wine and various other ingredients.

Punch Aboard Drunk.

Punch House Tavern where punch is sold.

Punch in the Mouth Strong drink of liquor.

Pungy Drunk.

Punish To drink all or a good part of bottle.

Punk Stuff Inferior liquor.

Punt Indentation at the base of some wine bottles, originally placed there for collecting the lees.

Puppy, Good Conditioned as a Drunk.

Purko Beer.

Purl Mixed drink made with hot ale, sugar, and infusion of wormwood. Popular during the eighteenth and nineteenth centuries. Often taken in the morning to produce an appetite.

Pussyfoot Prohibitionist.

Put a Few Bolsters back of the Bar To drink liquor.

Put a Full Cargo Aboard To get very drunk.

Put Away To drink liquor.

Put in Cold Storage To drink liquor.

Put it Down To drink liquor.

Put It where the Flies Won't Get It To drink liquor.

Put It where the Whale Put Jonah To drink liquor.

Put on the Drunk Act To get drunk.

Put the Make on *Same as* Panhandle.
Put to Bed with a Shovel Very drunk.
Put Your Name in the Pot Invitation to Drink.
Putrid Drunk.
Putting on the Rollers Drinking liquor.
Putt-putt Small motor boat used for smuggling liquor.
Pye-eyed Drunk.

Q

Quart bottle.

Q-F Quantity-frequency, a sociological indicant of drinking behavior.

Q-F-V Quantity-frequency-volume, a sociological indicant of drinking behavior.

Q.T. Illegal bar.

Quaff To drink the entire contents of a glass at one time.

Quarrelsome Drunk.

Queer Drunk.

Queer Joint Bar catering primarily to homosexuals.

Queered Drunk.

Quencher Drink of whiskey.

Quick Age To treat moonshine so that it has the appearance of aged whiskey by adding oak chips.

Quick One Drink to be consumed in haste.

Quiet One Private or surreptitious drink.

Quill Straw used to sample the distillate in a moonshiner's still as it is being produced.

Quilted Drunk.

R

Rabbit-footin *Same as* Piggy-back Doubling.

Race Pursuit of a moonshiner by a Treasury agent.

Rack To drain wine from one cask into another in order to remove the sediment.

Racked, Racked Up Drunk.

Racket Drinking spree.

Raddled Drunk.

Radiator Fluid Fluid containing isopropyl alcohol consumed when money for beverage alcohol cannot be obtained.

Rag Water Gin.

Ragged Drunk.

Railroad Whiskey Cheap wine.

Rainwater Madeira.

Raised Drunk.

Raised his Monuments Drunk.

Rammaged Drunk.

Rampage Very drunk.

Rams Delirium Tremens.

Randan Drinking spree.

Rantan Drinking spree.

Rat Bootlegger who carries liquor on his person.

Rat Hole Bar catering to a low-class clientele.

Rat in Trouble Drunk.

Rat Poison Inferior liquor.

Rat Race Alcoholism.

Rat Trap *Same as* Rat Hole.

Rats Delirium Tremens.

Rattle Belly Pop Mixture of lemonade and whiskey.

Rattle-blank-pop *Same as* Rattle Belly Pop.

Rattled Drunk.

Rat-track Whiskey Cheap liquor.

Ratty Drunk.

Raunchy Drunk.

Raw Undiluted whiskey.

Rawniel Beer.

Razors Strong liquor.

Razzee Drinking spree.

Razzle Dazzle Drinking spree.

Razzle-dazzled Drunk.

Reaches Vomiting produced by excessive drinking without eating.

Ready Drunk.

Real A. V. Liquor manufactured prior to Volstead Act. Good quality liquor.

Real Goods Bottled in bond liquor.

Real McCoy Bottled in bond liquor.

Real Stuff Good quality liquor.

Real Thing Bottled in bond liquor.

Really Gassed Very drunk.

Really Got a Load Very drunk.

Really Lit up Very drunk.

Really Soused Very drunk.

Really Tied One on Very drunk.

Rectified 1. Whiskey with additives blended into it to give it color and flavoring. 2. Concentrated by distillation, usually a second distillation.

Red Cheap wine.

Red Disturbance Whiskey.

Red-eye Cheap whiskey.

Red-eye Sour Whiskey and lemon.

Red Fustian Red wine.

Red Ink Red wine.

Red Liquor Strong liquor.

Red Nugget Illegal bar.

Red Onion *Same as* Red Nugget.

Red Ribbon Brandy.

Red Ruin Strong whiskey.

Red Tape Gin.

Red Tea Liquor.

Redistilled Alky Denatured alcohol.

Reeb Beer.

Reeking Drunk.

Reeling Drunk.

Reely Drunk.

Ree-raw Drunk.

Refresh the Inner Man To have a drink.

Refresher Drink taken as a stimulant.

Refreshery A bar.

Rehoboam Large wine bottle with capacity of six ordinary bottles.

Relaxed Drunk.

Religion, Got Given up drinking alcohol.

Religious Drunk.

Relished All Waters Heavy drinker.

Repeal Annulment of Prohibition.

Repeal Milk Liquor.

Reposer Nightcap.

Rerun Denatured alcohol.

Rerun Alky Reclaimed denatured alcohol.

Rescue Station Liquor store.

Rest, At Drunk.

Retsina Greek wine flavored with pine resin.

Revelation A drink.

Revenooer U.S. treasury revenue agent.

Revenuer *Same as* Revenooer.

Reverent Potent.

Reviver Drink of liquor.

Revved Up Mildly drunk.

Rhum Rum.

Ribbon Gin.

Rich Drunk.

Ride the Choo-choo Abstain from drinking.

Ride the Train Abstain from drinking.

Ride the Wagon Abstain from drinking.

Riding out of Town with Nothing but a Head Day after a drinking spree.

Rig Moonshiner's distillation equipment.

Rigid Drunk.

Rile To give liquor a turgid appearance.

Rileyed Drunk.

Rim Rams *Same as* Rams.

Rinse 1. Liquor. 2. To take a drink.

Rinser To drink to rinse food down.

Rip Drinking spree.

Ripe Drunk.

Ripped Very drunk.

Roaring Drunk Drunk and very boisterous.

Roasted Drunk.

Roasting Ear Wine Potent moonshine whiskey.

Robbing the Robbers To steal from those who rob drunks.

Rob-pot Drunkard.

Rocks Ice cubes.

Rocky Drunk.

Roll To go through a man's pockets while he is drunk.

Rolling Drunk Very drunk.

Rookus Juice Liquor.

Roostered Drunk.

Rorty Drunk.

Rose Red table wine partially fermented with grape skins.

Rose-colored glasses Glasses in which alcohol is served.

Rosin Alcohol given to musicians at a party.

Rosined Drunk.

Rosy 1. Drunk. 2. Wine.

Rosy About the Gills 1. *Same as* Rosy. 2. Flushed as a result of drinking.

Rot Gut 1. Bad liquor. 2. Wood alcohol.

Rotten Drunk.

Rotto Poor quality liquor.

Rouge Wine.

Round Drinks consumed by members of a group at the same time.

Rouse 1. Drunken party. 2. Large glass of some alcoholic beverage.

Rouser Drink taken as a stimulant.

Row Drunken frolic.

Rowing Men Group of drunkards.

Rowse *Same as* Rouse.

Royal Drunk.

Royal Bob Gin.

Royal Geneva Gin.

Royal Poverty Gin.

Rubber Drink Large glass of alcohol.

Rubbing alcohol Isopropyl alcohol used externally for medicinal purposes. Sometimes resorted to by destitute alcoholics.

Rubby-dubby Rubbing alcohol.

Ruby Wine.

Rudder, Lost his Drunk.

Ruin Inferior gin.

Rum 1. Alcohol beverage made from sugar cane. Contains a minimum of 80 proof alcohol. 2. Any type of liquor.

Rum Bag A drunkard.

Rum Baron Liquor magnate.

Rum Begrudged Rum that has been watered down.

Rum Beak Judge who could be bribed not to prosecute liquor smugglers.

Rum Bing A bar.

Rum Blossom Eruption of pimples on the nose.

Rum-bottle Drunken sailor.

Rum Bud Growth on the tip of the nose resulting from heavy drinking.

Rum Dumb 1. A drunkard. 2. Slow-witted from drinking too much rum. 3. Drunk.

Rum Fit Delirium Tremens.

Rum Fleet Fleet of boats smuggling illegal liquor.

Rum Head Heavy drinker.

Rum Hole Bar catering to low-class clientele.

Rum Hound *Same as* Rum Head.

Rum Jockey Heavy drinker.

Rum Mill A bar.

Rum Nose *Same as* Rum Bud.

Rum Pot A drunkard.

Rum Racket Business involving manufacture, sale, or distribution of illegal liquor.

Rum Ring Association of persons involved in the (usually illegal) sale of liquor.

Rum Row Line of liquor ships outside the U.S. territorial waters.

Rum Sick Experiencing a hangover.

Rum Soak A drunkard.

Rum Sucker A drunkard.

Rum Up To take a drink.

Rumbo Punch made with rum.

Rumbooze Rum.

Rumbose Wine.

Rumbowling Liquor.

Rumbullion Liquor made from rum and molasses.

Rumfustian Popular drink in England and colonies during eighteenth century. Made by pouring well-beaten eggs into beer, stirring, adding gin, and then adding boiling sherry.

Rumland The realm of liquor dealers and drinkers.

Rummed Drunk.

Rummer 1. Drinking spree. 2. A large glass for beer.

Rummied Drunk.

Rummy A drunkard.

Rummy Distiller Rum Baron.

Rummy Hound One who drinks large amounts of alcohol.

Rummy Nose Red nose associated with chronic, heavy drinking.

Rumrun Route through which liquor is smuggled.

Rumrunner Liquor smuggler.

Run 1. *Same as* Rum Run. 2. Completed distillation of moonshine whiskey.

Run Goods Smuggled liquor.

Run Out To finish distilling moonshine whiskey.

Runner One who transports moonshine from the moonshiner to the traffiker.

Running Hot Alcohol vapor passed too quickly through the still's condenser during production of moonshine whiskey.

Running the Mail Smuggling whiskey to soldiers in army forts.

Rush the Can To buy beer in pails to consume elsewhere.

Rush the Growler *Same as* Rush the Can.

Rye Distilled alcohol beverage made by fermenting rye.

Rye Sap Liquor.

Rye-soaked Drunk.

Rye Whiskey Whiskey distilled from grain containing at least 51 percent rye.

S

Saccharometer Instrument for measuring sugar content in wine and beer.

Saccharomyces cerevisiae Yeast stain used in fermenting wine and beer.

Sack Sherry.

Sack-posset Popular drink in England and the colonies during the early 1600s. Made with sack, ale, cream, eggs, and seasonings mixed together and boiled for several hours. Served at weddings, christenings, and parties.

Sail a Clear Sea To abstain from drinking.

Saint Martin's Evil Drunkenness.

Saint Patrick Whiskey.

Saint Patrick's Well *Same as* Saint Patrick.

Sake Japanese rice wine.

Sally Salvation Army.

Sally Stiff Salvation Army member.

Saloon Bar or tavern where drinks are served at tables.

Saloonist Owner of a saloon.

Saloonkeeper *Same as* Saloonist.

Salted Drunk.

Salted Down Drunk.

Salteur Liquor Diluted alcohol sold to Indians.

Salubrious Drunk.

Sample A drink.

Sample Room A bar.

Sampson Popular drink in United States during the eighteenth century. Made with rum and cider.

Sangaree, Sangry Sangria.

Sangria Red wine to which fruit juice has been added.

Santa Fe Express Wine to which codeine has been added.

Sap Alcohol.

Sap Happy Drunk.

Sapped Drunk.

Sappy Drunk.

Satin Gin.

Saturated Drunk.

Saturday Night Bottles Rum ration given to sailors after they had caught a whale.

Saturday Night Drinker One who drinks heavily only on weekends.

Sauce Liquor.

Sauce, On the Drinking alcohol regularly.

Sauced Drunk.

Sauterne Sweet white table wine.

Sawed Drunk.

Scalding Adding boiling water to cornmeal to begin the fermenting process.

Scammered Drunk.

Scamper Juice Poor-quality alcohol.

Scatter Illegal bar.

Schicker Drunk.

Schizzed Out Drunk.

Schlitzed Drunk.

Schlockered Drunk.

Schnapps Any liquor with a high alcohol content, such as brandy, gin, or whiskey.

Schnockered Drunk.

Schnoggered Drunk.

Schnozzle too deeply To drink too much.

Schooner 1. Large glass for beer. 2. Place where alcohol is sold illegally.

Schooner of Suds Large glass of beer.

Scofflaw One who derided the Prohibition Amendment.

Scooch Rum.

Scoop 1. Glass of beer. 2. Drunk.

Scoop, On the Drinking excessively.

Scooped Drunk.

Scorched Drunk.

Scorched liquor Whiskey made from mash that has been scorched from being on the bottom of the fermenter.

Scorching Fluid Liquor.

Scorpion Bible Cheap whiskey.

Scot Ale Private drinking party of those who brought their own ale.

Scotch Whiskey from Scotland.

Scotchem Popular early American drink made with apple jack, boiling water, and a dash of mustard. Mostly consumed in New Jersey.

Scowrer A drunkard.

Scrambled Drunk.

Scrambled Egg A drunkard.

Scrap Iron Bootleg drink combining alcohol and mothballs.

Scratched 1. Drunk. 2. No longer having credit at a bar or liquor store.

Scraunched Drunk.

Screaming Drunk.

Screaming Abdams Delirium Tremens.

Screaming Drunk Drunk and argumentative.

Screaming Meanies 1. Experiencing symptoms of hangover. 2. Delirium Tremens.

Screetching Drunk.

Screw A drink.

Screwed Drunk.

Screwy Drunk.

Scronched Drunk.

Scrooched Drunk.

Scrooped Drunk.

Scuds Beer.

Scuttle A large beer mug.

Scuttle Butt A bar.

Scuttle of Suds Large glass of beer.

Seafaring Drunk.

Sealed Quart Standard measure for ale containing an "ale-taster's" mark.

Seasick Drunk.

Second Sugar To add sugar to mash already used so that a second distillation of moonshine whiskey can be made.

Second-Hand Drunk To become drunk from inhaling the breath of someone who has been drinking.

Sediment Solid insoluble material which falls to the bottom of a cask or wine bottle after it has been standing for some time.

See a Man, To To drink at a bar.

See Double Impaired vision from drinking too much.

See Double and Feel Single *Same as* See Double.

Seeing a Flock of Moons Drunk.

Seeing Bats Drunk.

Seeing Bears Drunk.

Seeing Double Drunk.

Seeing Elephants Drunk.

Seeing Pink Elephants Delirium Tremens.

Seeing Snakes Delirium Tremens.

Seeing the Devil Drunk.

Seeing Two Moons Drunk.

Seek a Clove To take a drink.

Sell One's Senses Drunk.

Sensation Quart of gin.

Sent Drunk.

Sentiment Sediment.

Sentimental Water Liquor.

September Morn Undiluted drink of liquor.

Serpentina Condensing coil in a still.

Serum Alcohol.

Served, Served Up Drunk.

Service wine Wine made from mountain ash berries.

Set *Same as* Still.

Set 'em up To pour a drink.

Set Up 1. Equipment for preparing drinks. 2. To pay for drinks for others. 3. Drunk.

Setting-up Exercise Drinking.

Settler Final drink before retiring.

Sewed, Sewed Up Drunk.

Sewer Cheap drinking place.

Sewer Pipe A drunkard.

Shack 1. Large beer mug. 2. Enclosure in which a moonshiner's still is hidden.

Shagged Drunk.

Shaggy Drunk.

Shake a Cloth To take a drink.

Shake-em-up White wine and lemon juice.

Shake Tail Cocktail.

Shake Up Cocktail.

Shaker A drunkard.

Shakes Delirium Tremens.

Shaky Experiencing hangover.

Sham Champagne.

Shammy Champagne.

Shandy-gaff Mixture of ale and ginger beer.

Shant A drink.

Shave the guts To take a drink.

Shaved Drunk.

Shebeen Illegal bar.

Shed a Tear To take a drink.

Sheepdip Inferior liquor.

Sheepherder's Delight Cheap whiskey.

Shell *Same as* Bootlegger.

Shellac Inferior liquor.

Shellack the tonsils Take a drink.

Shellacked Drunk.

Sherry Sweet fortified wine.

Shews his Hobnails Drunk.

Shick Drunk.

Shicked Drunk.

Shicker 1. A drunkard. 2. Drunk.

Shickered Drunk.

Shikker Drunk.

Shikkered Drunk.

Shim-shams Delirium Tremens.

Shindy Drinking spree.

Shine Illicitly make whiskey. Moonshine.

Shined Drunk on moonshine.

Shiner 1. Moonshiner. 2. Bootlegger.

Shinery Illegal bar.

Shinny 1. Drunk. 2. Potent moonshine whiskey.

Shipwrecked Drunk.

Shit-faced Drunk.

Shitter Drinking spree.

Shitty Drunk.

Shock Joint 1. Bar. 2. Illegal bar.

Shoe Pinches Him Drunk.

Shoe Polish Whiskey.

Shoe Polish Shop Place where alcohol is sold illegally.

Shoot 1. To add alcohol to nonalcoholic drinks. 2. To take a drink.

Shoot One *Same as* Shoot.

Shoot the Boot Drinking game in which a dirty sneaker is filled with beer and the contents are consumed.

Short Unadulterated.

Short One A small drink.

Short Pull A small drink; sometimes used in reference to a drink from a flask.

Shorty 1. Liquor. 2. Drunk.

Shot 1. Drink of undiluted whiskey. 2. Drunk.

Shot and a Beer Whiskey followed by beer.

Shot and Beer Joint A bar.

Shot Beer Beer to which other more concentrated forms of alcohol are added.

Shot full of Holes Drunk.

Shot Glass Premeasured glass for serving liquor.

Shot in the Arm A drink.

Shot in the Head Drunk.

Shot in the Mouth Drunk.

Shot in the Neck Drunk.

Shot in the Wrist Drunk.

Shot of Moon Drink of moonshine liquor.

Shot under the Wing Drunk.

Shot Up Drunk.

Shoulder, Burnt his Drunk.

Shout 1. Take a drink. 2. Payment for a round of drinks.

Showing his Booze Drunk.

Showing his Drinks Drunk.

Showing It Drunk.

Shows his Hob-nails Drunk.

Shrub Generic term for alcohol beverage made from fruit juice.

Shupper Large beer mug.

Shut Off To refuse to serve a customer any more drinks.

Sick Experiencing hangover.

Sick Wine Wine.

Side-pocket Place where liquor is sold illegally.

Silk Stocking Chapter of Alcoholics Anonymous in which most members are socially well-to-do.

Silken Twine Wine.

Sillabub *Same as* Syllabub.

Silly Drunk.

Silly Drunk Drunk.

Silly Milk Alcohol.

Simon Pure Bottled in bond liquor.

Single Beer Inferior beer.

Single Broth Inferior beer.

Single One Inferior liquor.

Singlings First distillate product during distillation of alcohol.

Sinker A drunkard.

Siphon Take a drink.

Sipter A heavy drinker.

Sissy Beer Beer with a low alcohol content.

Sitting of the Bead The position of bubbles after a jar of moonshine whiskey has been shaken.

Six, Cup of Cup of beer.

Six Water Grog Diluted rum.

Sizzled Drunk.

Skate 1. Drinking spree. 2. One who is on a drinking spree.

Skated Drunk.

Skates, Got on his On a drinking spree.

Skee Liquor.

Skid Row Run-down urban area inhabited by derelicts and destitute alcoholics.

Skid Row Bum Alcoholic on skid row.

Skikker *Same as* Shicker.

Skin-disease Inferior beer.

Skinful 1. Drunk. 2. Having consumed a large amount of liquor.

Skink 1. Drink of liquor. 2. To draw or pour out liquor.

Skinker One who dispenses ale or owns a tavern.

Skit Beer.

Skoal Drinking toast.

Skull Dragging Begging for drinks in a bar.

Skull Varnish Whiskey.

Skunk Drunk Drunk.

Skunked Drunk.

Skunky Drunk.

Sky Whiskey.

Sky Blue Gin.

Slanted Drunk.

Slathered Drunk.

Slave of the Beast A drunkard.

Sleeve-button Drunk.

Slewed Drunk.

Slewy Drunk.

Slick Drunk.

Slight Sensation Liquor.

Sling Drink made with various types of liquors but usually gin, water, ice, and bitters.

Slinger One who drinks in the morning.

Slip To resume drinking after an alcoholic's period of abstinence.

Slippery Drunk.

Slipping Drunk.

Slipslap Weak, inferior liquor.

Slipslop Weak, inferior liquor.

Slobber Box *Same as* Thump Keg.

Slobbered Drunk.

Slop 1. Liquor. 2. *Same as* Spent Beer.

Slop Down To take a drink.

Slop Up To drink to the point of intoxication.

Slop-dash Weak, inferior liquor.

Slopped Drunk.

Slopped Over *Same as* Slopped.

Slopped to the Ears *Same as* Slopped.

Slopped to the Gills *Same as* Slopped.

Slopping Back Reusing boiled mash to scald a new batch rather than using boiling water in making moonshine.

Slopping Up On a drinking spree.

Sloppy Drunk.

Slops Inferior beer.

Slosh Alcohol.

Sloshed Drunk.

Sloud Drunk.

Slough up To take a drink.

Sloughed Drunk.

Slubber Heavy drinker.

Slued Drunk.

Slug A drink.

Slug, Fire a To take a drink.

Slug of Blue Fish Hooks Drink of cider.

Slugged Drunk.

Sluice 1. A drink. 2. To take a drink.

Sluice your Bolt Take a drink.

Slumgullion Weak, inferior liquor.

Slush Weak, inferior liquor.

Slush Up To drink to the point of intoxication.

Slushed Drunk.

Slusher A drunkard.

Smack Alcoholic content or reaction.

Small Beer 1. Weak beer; beer of inferior quality and taste. 2. Second extract from fermented malt, taken after the ale has been drained away.

Small Cheque Small drink.

Smaller Regular-sized drink.

Smash 1. Generic term for an alcohol beverage like a julep, except with fewer ingredients. 2. Wine.

Smash a Brandy Peg To take a drink.

Smashed Drunk.

Smeared Drunk.

Smell Large glass of beer.

Smells of the Cork Drunk.

Smile 1. Small drink. 2. To take a drink.

Smiler 1. One who drinks often. 2. Full glass.

Smilo Alcoholic cider.

Smitten by the Grape Drunk on wine.

Smoke 1. Alcohol. 2. Rye.

Smoke House A bar.

Smoked Drunk.

Snack Bar Bar that also serves light lunches.

Snackered Drunk.

Snake Whiskey.

Snake Head Whiskey Cheap whiskey.

Snake in the Boots Delirium Tremens.

Snake Juice Poor-quality whiskey.

Snake Medicine Liquor.

Snake Pit Bar with a bad reputation.

Snake Poison *Same as* Snake Juice.

Snake Water Whiskey.

Snakebite Medicine Whiskey.

Snakes Delirium Tremens.

Snap Neck Brandy.

Snapped 1. Drunk. 2. Arrested for public drunkenness.

Sneak Bottle 1. Bottle of Sneaky Peat. 2. Bottle that one drinks in secret.

Sneak Drinker One who drinks surreptitiously.

Sneakeasy Illegal bar.

Sneaker 1. Motorboat used to smuggle liquor. 2. Still.

Sneakie Illegal bar.

Sneaky-Pete 1. Cheap alcohol consumed by skid row alcoholics. 2. Cheap wine. 3. Marihuana mixed with wine.

Sneaky-Pete Pounder Experiencing hangover after drinking too much wine.

Sneaky Peter One who drinks cheap wine.

Snicker Drinking cup.

Sniff A drink.

Sniff the Cork To take a drink.

Snifter 1. Small drink of liquor. 2. Small short-stemmed glass.

Snip Small glass or drink of liquor.

Snit Small glass kept by a bartender beneath the bar.

Snockered Drunk.

Snooted Drunk.

Snootful 1. Drunk. 2. Figuratively having consumed enough liquor to fill one from the feet up to the nose.

Snootful, Had a Drunk.

Snootful, Have a To have a drink.

Snopsy Gin.

Snort 1. A drink. 2. To take a drink.

Snorter 1. A drink. 2. A drunkard.

Snotted Drunk.

Snowballs Large bubbles produced during fermentation.

Snozzle Wobbles To be hungover.

Snozzled Drunk.

Snubbed Drunk.

Snuffy Drunk.

Snug Drunk.

Soak 1. A drunkard. 2. Drinking spree. 3. A drink.

Soak your Chaffer To take a drink.

Soaked Drunk.

Soaked his Face Drunk.

Soaked the Mill Sold all of one's possessions in getting money to buy liquor.

Soaked to the Gills Drunk.

Soaken Drunk.

Soaker A drunkard.

Soaking Wet Anti-prohibitionist.

Soapy-eyed Drunk.

Sobbed Drunk.

Sober Not under the influence of alcohol.

Sober as a Buck Shad Sober.

Sober as a Church Sober.

Sober as a Deacon Sober.

Sober as a Judge Sober.

Sober as a Shoemaker Sober.

Sober Side of the Bar The side of the bar occupied by the bartender.

Sobering-up Station Place where drunks are taken to sober up overnight rather than a jail.

Sobriety 1. Temperate in drinking. 2. Abstinent.

Social Drinking Drinking in moderation, usually in the company of others.

Social Lubricant Liquor.

Sock Alcoholic content or reaction.

Socked Drunk.

Sod A drunkard.

Soda Pop Moon Moonshine bottled in discarded soft-drink bottles.

Soda Water Water with carbon dioxide.

Sodden Drunk.

Sodden Bum A drunkard.

Soft 1. Not containing alcohol. 2. Drunk.

Soggy Drunk.

Sold his Senses Drunk.

Solitary Drinker One who drinks alone rather than with others.

Solomon, As wise as Drunk.

Something Liquor.

Something Damp A drink.

Something on the Hip Pocket flask for liquor.

Something on the Saddle Pocket flask for liquor.

Something Short Small glass or drink of liquor.

Sommelier Wine waiter.

Soother Liquor.

Soothing Syrup Liquor.

Sop A drunkard.

Sopped Drunk.

Sopping Drunk.

Sopping Wet 1. *Same as* Sopping. 2. Anti-prohibitionist.

Soppy Drunk.

Sore-Footed Drunk.

Sorrow Drowner Liquor.

Soshed Drunk.

S.O.T. "Son of intemperance"; heavy drinker.

Sot A drunkard.

Sot in the Main Brace To get drunk.

Sotted Drunk.

Sottish Confused by drinking too much.

Sottishness Drunken stupidity.

Sotto Drunk.

Sotto Voce Parlor Illegal bar.

Sound Card Heavy drinker.

Soupy Drunk to the point of sickness.

Sour Generic term for an alcohol beverage and the skin of a lemon placed in a glass.

Sour Beer Vinegar made from beer.

Sour Mash Method of producing whiskey in which the corn and rye mixture is scalded with a previously discarded distillate.

Souse 1. A drunkard. 2. A drinking spree.

Soused Drunk.

Soused to the Ears Very drunk.

Soused to the Gills Very drunk.

Southern Fried Drunk.

Sow Drunk Very drunk.

Sozzled Drunk.

Sozzly Drunk.

Spark in the Throat Thirst for a drink.

Sparkle Champagne.

Sparkling Wine Wine fermented twice and heavily carbonated as a result.

Sparred Drunk.

Sparrow Inferior whiskey.

Speak Speakeasy.

Speakeasy Place where alcohol is sold illegally.

Speaketeer Speakeasy racketeer.

Speaks Speakeasies.

Speared Drunk.

Speck Small glass of liquor.

Speck Bum Destitute drunkard who lives by scrounging for food in garbage cans.

Speechless Drunk.

Speedball Adulterated glass of wine.

Spent Beer Distillate remaining after the alcohol has been removed from the mash.

Spent Mash *Same as* Spent Beer.

Spiffed Drunk.

Spiffled Drunk.

Spiflicated Drunk.

Spigot-Bigot Prohibitionist.

Spike To add liquor to another beverage.

Spiked Beer Beer to which other kinds of alcohol have been added.

Spile Peg at the end of a cask of liquor.

Spile Hole The hole at the end of a cask of liquor.

Spirits Alcohol.

Spit White Drink a lot.

Splash A drinking spree.

Splash Can *Same as* Thump Keg.

Splashed Drunk.

Spliced Drunk.

Splice the Main Brace To take a drink.

Splifficated Drunk.

Spliffo Drunk.

Split Small bottle of liquor, usually about a half pint.

Split a Few Seals To share a bottle.

Split Case Half case of beer, usually 12 bottles.

Sploshed Drunk.

Sponge 1. Heavy drinker. 2. To drink at someone else's cost.

Sponge Up To take a drink.

Sponge-eyed Drunk.

Sponge-headed Drunk.

Sportsman for Liquor Heavy drinker.

Spot 1. Illegal bar. 2. Place where liquor that had been smuggled was unloaded.

Spotty Drunk.

Sprang Alcohol.

Spree 1. Extended drinking binge. 2. A drink.

Spreed Drunk.

Spreester One who is on a spree.

Sprinkled Drunk.

Sprung Drunk.

Spumante Sparkling wine from Italy.

Spun-joint Place where home-spun is sold.

Squail A drink.

Squamed Drunk.

Squared Drunk.

Squashed Drunk.

Squeeze Methanol removed from parrafin by passing it through a stocking.

Squiffed Drunk.

Squiffy Drunk.

Squirrel Moonshine.

Squirrel Cage Alcoholism.

Squirrel Dew *Same as* Squirrel.

Squirrelly Drunk.

Squished Drunk.

S.R.D. Service Rum Diluted, initials imprinted on rum jars.

Staff Naked Gin.

Stagger Juice Whiskey.

Stagger Soup Liquor.

Stagger Water Liquor.

Staggerish Drunk.

Staggers Wobbly drunk.

Staggery Drunk.

Stale Drunk 1. Perpetually drunk. 2. Drunkard who has been on a prolonged drinking spree.

Stand To pay for everyone's drink.

Stand One against the Bar To pay for everyone's drinks.

Stand Sam To pay for everyone's drinks.

Starched Drunk.

Starchy Drunk.

Stark Drunk Drunk.

Starter First drink in the morning.

Starting to Feel Good Beginning to feel euphoric from alcohol.

Starting to Feel Rosy *Same as* Starting to Feel Good.

Starting to Glow *Same as* Starting to Feel Good.

Stash Raw materials for making moonshine or moonshine itself that has been hidden.

Station Drink Whiskey.

Steadier Strong drink.

Steady Drunk.

Steam beer Beer fermented at a very high temperature causing the container to build up considerable pressure. Heavily hopped with a bitter taste.

Steamed Drunk.

Steeped Drunk.

Steer Joint Store that directs one to an illegal bar.

Stem *Same as* Panhandle.

Step Up Add liquor to another beverage.

Sterno Commercial item containing methanol in paraffin.

Stew 1. Alcohol. 2. A destitute alcoholic.

Stew Bum A drunkard.

Stewed Drunk.

Stewed Fruit A drunkard.

Stewed to the Gills Very drunk.

Stewie A drunkard.

Stick l. Dash of spirits. 2. A bar.

Stick, Behind the Working as a bartender.

Stick'em up To pay for everyone's drink.

Sticked Drunk.

Stiff 1. Drunk. 2. A drunkard.

Stiff as a Carp Drunk.

Stiff as a Goat Drunk.

Stiff as a Plank Drunk.

Stiff as a Ramrod Drunk.

Stiff as a Ring-bolt Drunk.

Stiff Blade Heavy drinker.

Stiff Drink Strong alcohol drink.

Stiff Glass Strong drink of liquor.

Stiffed Drunk.

Stiffo Drunk.

Still 1. Apparatus for producing moonshine whiskey. 2. Quiet drunkard.

Still beer Initial part of distilled moonshine whiskey that contains a low percentage of alcohol.

Stillage *Same as* Spent Beer.

Stiller Distiller.

Stillin' Making Moonshine.

Stimulated Drunk.

Stinger Whiskey and soda.

Stingo Potent liquor.

Stinkarooed Drunk.

Stinking Very drunk.

Stinking Drunk Very drunk.

Stinko Very drunk.

Stirrup Cup Parting drink.

Stitched Drunk.

Stocked Up Drunk.

Stoked Drunk.

Stolled Drunk.

Stone Blind Very drunk.

Stone Cold Drunk Drunk.

Stone Fence Popular drink during colonial period, made with cider, apple brandy, brown sugar, and spices.

Stone Sober Sober.

Stoned Very drunk.

Stoned out of his Mind Drunk.

Stone-wall Popular drink in U.S. during eighteenth century, made with rum and cider.

Stonkered Very drunk.

Stoop, Stoup A drinking vessel.

Stout Dark, sweet beer with high hops content.

Stozzled Drunk.

Straight 1. Alcohol. 2. Undiluted.

Straight Corn Moonshine whiskey made from corn alone. No sugar is added and no attempt is made to adulterate it in any way.

Straight Drinking Drinking at a bar instead of at a table.

Straight Stuff Liquor.

Straight Up Drink served without ice.

Straight whiskey Whiskey made from grain mash, distilled at no more than 80 percent alcohol, and aged for at least two years.

Straighten Out To stop drinking.

Straightener First drink in the morning.

Strengthy Potent.

Strike-me-dead Inferior beer.

Strip-me-naked Gin.

Strip Stamp Government stamp placed over the neck and cap of a bottle of alcohol showing that a tax has been paid on it.

Striped Drunk.

Strong High alcohol content.

Strong Waters Distilled spirits.

Strunt Strong liquor.

Stubbed Drunk.

Stube Bar that also serves light lunches.

Stuccoed Drunk.

Studding Sails Out Drunk.

Stuff Liquor.

Stuff that Cheers Liquor.

Stumble Bum Destitute alcoholic.

Stumble Drunk Drunk and unable to walk.

Stump Likker, Liquor Moonshine.

Stump Whiskey Moonshine.

Stung Drunk.

Stunko Drunk.

Stunned Drunk.

Stupefied Drunk.

Stupid Drunk.

Submarine Distillation apparatus with large tubs used as stills.

Subtle as a Fox Heavy drinker.

Suck 1. To take a drink. 2. Any alcoholic beverage.

Suck some Corn Juice *Same as* Suck.

Suck the Bottle *Same as* Suck.

Suck the Monkey *Same as* Suck.

Suck the Spigot *Same as* Suck.

Suck Your Face *Same as* Suck.

Sucked Drunk.

Sucker A drunkard.

Suckerdom Realm of drinkers.

Sucking the monkey Taking wine secretly from a cask.

Suck-spiggot A drunkard.

Sucky Drunk.

Suds Beer.

Suds, A Little in the Drunk.

Suds, In the Drunk.

Suds Factory A brewery.

Suds Jerker Bartender.

Suds Joint A bar mainly serving beer.

Suds Slinger Bartender.

Sudsery Beer parlor.

Suet Liquor.

Suffer it Out Go through withdrawal from alcohol.

Sugar Jack 100 proof whiskey made with a small amount of corn and a large amount of sugar.

Sugar Liquor *Same as* Sugar Jack.

Sugar mash Concentrated sugar solution added to corn in the fermenting process for moonshine whiskey.

Sugar the Kidney To take a drink.

Sugarhead Moonshine whiskey made with a very high sugar content and known to cause painful headaches in consumers.

Suit and Cloth 1. Any agreeable liquor. 2. Store of brandy.

Sun, Been in the Drunk.

Sun in the Eyes Drunk.

Sun over the Fore-yard Drunk.

Sundowner Drink taken before retiring for the night.

Super-Charged Drunk.

Swack A drink.

Swacked Drunk.

Swacko Drunk.

Swallowed a Tavern Token Drunk.

Swamped Drunk.

Swamper Bartender.

Swamproot Potent moonshine whiskey.

Swankey Inferior beer.

Swaper Barroom porter.

Swatched Drunk.

Swatted Drunk.

Swattled Drunk.

Swazzled Drunk.

Sweat *Same as* Bulldog.

Sweat it Out To go through withdrawal from alcohol.

Sweats Distress experienced during alcohol withdrawal.

Sweet Wine with a high sugar content.

Sweet Lightnin' Moonshine whiskey to which sweeteners have been added.

Sweet Lucy Port wine.

Sweet Mash Method of producing bourbon in which fresh yeast is added to each mixture of corn and rye.

Sweet Waters Illegal liquor made from the residue of a cider press.

Swell Head A drunkard.

Swicky Whiskey.

Swig 1. Popular drink in England during the eighteenth century. Made from spiced ale, wine, and toast. 2. Large amount of alcohol consumed in one long swallow.

Swig at the Halyards Drink taken in secret by a sailor.

Swig Up To take a drink.

Swigged Drunk.

Swigger A drunkard.

Swiggle To take a drink.

Swiggled Drunk.

Swiggling Drinking.

Swill l. Alcohol. 2. To guzzle.

Swill-belly A drunkard.

Swilled, Swilled Up Drunk.

Swiller A drunkard.

Swill-pot A drunkard.

Swine Drunk Moderately drunk.

Swiney Drunk.

Swinnied Drunk.

Swiped Drunk.

Swiper A drunkard.

Swipes Inferior beer.

Swipey Slightly drunk.

Swish-swash Inferior beer.

Switchel Weak alcoholic drink popular in New England during colonial period. Made with cider, water, and spices.

Switchy Drunk.

Swively Drunk.

Swizzle 1. To drink alcohol. 2. Beer.

Swizzle Guts A drunkard.

Swizzle Nick A drunkard.

Swizzle Stick Stirrer for mixing ingredients in alcoholic beverages.

Swizzled Drunk.

Swizzy Rum.

Swozzled Drunk.

Syllabub Popular drink in England and the United States during the eighteenth century. Made with wine and milk or cream to which sugar and sometimes spices were added.

Synergistic Combination of drug agents which results in a greater effect than that which would be produced by each drug agent alone.

T

Tab Bill at a bar or liquor store.

Table wine Wine consumed during meals.

Tacky Drunk.

Take a Cup too much To drink to the point of intoxication.

Take a (One's) Drop To take a drink.

Take a Jolt To take a drink.

Take a Nip To take a drink.

Take a Pull To take a drink.

Take a Shot To take a drink.

Take a Shot in the Arm To take a drink.

Take a Shove in the Guts To take a drink.

Take a Shove in the Mouth To take a drink.

Take a Slug To take a drink.

Take a Smell To take a drink.

Take a Sneak To take a drink without anyone noticing.

Take a Snifter To take a drink.

Take a Snort To take a drink at a bar.

Take a Wet To take a drink.

Take an Oath To take a drink.

Take More than You can Hold To drink to the point of intoxication.

Take on Fuel To drink a lot of alcohol.

Take One over the Eight To drink to the point of intoxication.

Take some Cheer To take a drink.

Take Something for the Stomach To take a drink.

Take the Pledge To declare that one will no longer drink alcoholic beverages.

Take your Medicine To take a drink.

Tangle Foot Bad liquor.

Tangle-footed Drunk.

Tangle Leg Alcohol.

Tangled Drunk.

Tangled-legged Drunk.

Tank 1. A drunkard. 2. Person with a large capacity for drinking. 3. Jail cell in which drunkards are kept overnight.

Tank Up To take a drink.

Tankard Drinking vessel with a handle.

Tanked, Tanked Up Drunk.

Tanned Drunk.

Tannin Substance in grape skin that gives wine an astringent taste.

Tap 1. A beer parlor. 2. Taproom.

Tap, On Beer served by draft rather than by bottle.

Taper Off Decrease one's alcohol intake.

Tapeteria *Same as* Tap.

Taplash Dregs from the bottom of a beer keg.

Taplash Wretched Drunk.

Tapped Drunk.

Tapped Out Drunk.

Tapped the Admiral Drunk.

Tap-shackled Drunk.

Taproom, Tap Room Place where draft beer is sold.

Tapster Bartender who pours beer for customers.

Tarantula-juice Potent liquor.

Tattooed Drunk.

Tavern Originally a place where wine was sold (in contrast to ale-house). No longer restricted to type of beverage served.

Taverner 1. Drunkard. One who spends a lot of time in a tavern. 2. Tavern owner.

Tead Drunk.

Tear Up To go on a drinking spree.

Tears of a Tankard Drops of good liquor.

Teed Drunk.

Teeth Under Drunk.

Teetotaler, T-totaler Abstainer from alcohol. From the repetition of the letter T in total, for emphasis.

Temperance Moderation, usually used in reference to alcohol.

Temperance Drink Nonalcoholic beverage.

Temperance Movement Political action movement seeking to ban alcohol consumption prior to World War I. Efforts resulted in Prohibition in the United States.

Temperance Pledge *See* Take the Pledge.

Temperance Society Group that restricts consumption of alcohol as part of its program, (e.g., Women's Christian Temperance Union).

Temperate Moderate in consumption of alcohol.

Temping Bottle Bottle for testing quality of moonshine by inspecting beads formed on the surface after contents have been shaken.

Temulent Drunk.

Temulentious Drunk.

Temulentive Drunk.

Tent Red wine from Spain. Term used during 1600s.

Tequila Liquor made from agave cactus. Popular drink in Mexico.

Thawed Drunk.

There Drunk.

Thick Head Drunkenness.

Thick-lipped Drunk.

Thick-tongued Drunk.

Third Party Payment Payment made to service provider, (e.g., doctor, hospital), from someone other than patient (e.g., insurance program, government) for all or part of service provided to patient.

Third Rail Potent whiskey.

Thirst-aid Station A bar.

Three Bricks Short of a Load Drunk.

Three Sheets to the Wind Drunk.

Three Sheets to the Wind and One Flapping Drunk.

Throw To empty the contents of a glass without pausing.

Throw a Wingding To go on a drinking spree.

Throw away the Cork To get drunk.

Thump Keg Keg located between the boiler and condenser of a moonshine still. Alcohol vapor passes through it but impurities condense inside and are drained off.

Thumped over the Head with Sampson's Jawbone Drunk.

Thumper *Same as* Thump Keg.

Tick *Same as* Tab.

Tickle-pitcher Drinking companion.

Tickler Small bottle of liquor.

Tiddled Drunk.

Tiddley Drunk.

Tiddy Drunk.

Tie One On To drink a lot of alcohol.

Tied One On Drank considerably and became intoxicated.

Tiff Alcohol.

Tiffed Drunk.

Tiffled Drunk.

Tiger Milk Potent alcoholic drink.

Tiger Piss Poor-quality beer.

Tiger Sweat Whiskey.

Tight Drunk.

Tight as a Brassier *Same as* Tight.

Tight as a Drum *Same as* Tight.

Tight as a Goat *Same as* Tight.

Tight as a Mink *Same as* Tight.

Tight as a Ten Day Drunk Very drunk.

Tight as a Tick *Same as* Tight.

Tight as the Bark on a Tree Same as Tight.

Tilted Drunk.

Tin Hats Drunk.

Tinned Drunk.

Tip To take a drink.

Tip Merry Drunk.

Tip Top Drunk.

Tip Top Tippler Drunk on champagne.

Tipium Grove Drunk.

Tipped Drunk.

Tipping Drunk.

Tipple To sip alcohol.

Tippler Drunkard.

Tippling Drunk.

Tipply Drunk.

Tippy Drunk.

Tipsification Drunkenness.

Tipsified Drunk.

Tipsify Intoxicate.

Tipsy Drunk.

Tired Drunk.

Titley Drinking spree.

Tittery Gin.

Toast 1. Invitation to drink to wish someone good health or fortune. 2. A drunkard.

Toast and Butter Drunkard.

Toasted Drunk.

Tod, Will you Invitation to drink.

Toddy, Hot Mixture of rum, whiskey, hot water, and various spices.

Toddy Blossom Eruption of pimples on the nose or face.

Tolerance Adaptation of the body to the point where more of a given drug is required to produce the same effect as when used originally.

Tom and Jerry Shop Low-class bar.

Tongue-tied Drunk.

Tonsil Paint Alcohol.

Tonsil Varnish Poor-quality liquor.

Tonsil Wash Liquor.

Tonsil Wash Emporium A bar.

Too Far North Drunk.

Took a Flip To have resumed drinking after a period of abstinence.

Toot l. A drink. 2. Drinking spree.

Top Heavy Drunk.

Top Loaded Drunk.

Top Off To finish drinking whatever remains in the glass.

Tope To drink heavily.

Toped Drunk.

Toper A drunkard.

Topped Drunk.

Toppled Very drunk.

Toppy Drunk.

Topsy Turvey Drunk.

Torn Up Drunk.

Torpedo Whiskey to which chloral hydrate has been added.

Torrid Drunk.

Toss To take a drink.

Tossed Drunk.

Tosspot A drunkard.

Tosticated Drunk.

Totalled Very drunk.

Touched Drunk.

Touched Off Drunk.

Tough as a Boiled Owl Belligerent as a result of drinking.

Toxed Drunk.

Toxic Poisonous.

Toxicated Drunk.

Toxy Drunk.

Traffiker Middleman in production and sale of moonshine who obtained moonshine from the runner and delivered it to the buyer.

Trammeled Drunk.

Trance, In a Drunk.

Translated Drunk.

Trashed Drunk.

Tremens Delirium tremens.

Tremor Involuntary trembling or shaking.

Tripping Drunk.

True Blew Heavy drinker.

Try a Smile, Will you? Invitation to drink.

Tubed Drunk.

Tumbled down the Sink Very drunk.

Tun Wine cask. Contains about 252 gallons.

Tune Up To take a drink.

Tuned Drunk.

Tuned Up Drunk.

Twelve Steps Twelve principles and rules underlying Alcoholics Anonymous.

Twenty-first Amendment Amendment to U.S. Constitution repealing prohibition.

Twisted Drunk.

Twister Drinking spree.

Two-fisted Drinker Heavy drinker who is able to drink a lot without becoming drunk.

Two Sheets to the Wind Slightly drunk. *See also* Three Sheets to the Wind.

U

Ugglies Delirium Tremens.

Ugly Drunk.

Ullage 1. Space between bottom of a cork or top of a cask and the top of the wine in a container. 2. Spoiled beer.

Ultra-dry Favoring Prohibition.

Umph An alcoholic.

Unalloyed Undiluted liquor.

Uncorked Drunk.

Uncorrupted Undiluted liquor.

Under Drunk.

Under Full Sail Drunk.

Under Full Steam Drunk.

Under the Influence Impaired by alcohol but not drunk.

Under the Table Drunk.

Under the Weather Drunk.

Underway Drunk.

Undiluted Undiluted or unadulterated liquor.

Unmarried *Same as* Undiluted.

Unsober Drunk.

Unsophisticated *Same as* Undiluted.

Untempered Undiluted liquor.

Up a Tree Drunk.

Up on Blocks Drunk.

Up the Bucket To take a drink.

Up the Pole Drunk.

Up to the Gills Drunk.

Upholster To become drunk.

Upholstered Drunk.

Uppercut Brandy.

Uppish Drunk.

Uprights Measures of liquor.

Upse-Dutch Strong beer imported from Holland.

Upse-freese Strong beer imported from Friesland.

Upsey Drunk.

Usisge beatha Whiskey.

Usquebaugh Whiskey.

V

Valiant Drunk.

Valley Tan Whiskey.

Varietal Wine named after the type of grape used to make it (in contrast to naming it after its native geographical area).

Varnish Inferior liquor.

Varnished Drunk.

Vat *Same as* Fermenter.

Veeno Wine.

Verder Rum and fruit drink popular in American colonies.

Vermouth Fortified wine infused with herbs. Taken alone or mixed with liquors such as gin.

Vim Alcoholic content or reaction.

Vinegar Originally sour wine.

Vineyard Field where grapes are grown.

Viniculture Cultivation of grapes.

Vino Wine.

Vinolence Drunkenness from too much wine.

Vinomania Uncontrollable craving for wine.

Vintage The year the grapes used to make a particular wine were harvested.

Vintner Wine merchant.

Virgin Glass Undiluted drink.

Virginia drams Brandy made from peaches, popular in the Southern American colonies.

Visne Mixture of brandy and wine.

Vitamin A Liquor.

Viticulture *Same as* Viniculture.

Vitriol Inferior liquor.

Vodka Liquor made from charcoal-filtered grain or potatoes to remove taste, aroma, and color.

Volstead Act 18th amendment to U.S. constitution prohibiting manufacture, distribution, and sale of alcohol.

Volstead Exile Liquor made before the Volstead Act took effect.

Volsteadian Prohibitionist.

Volsteadite Prohibitionist.

Vulcanized Drunk.

W

Wagon, On the No longer drinking.

Wagon Rider Abstainer.

Waker-upper First drink of the day.

Walking Whiskey Vat Heavy drinker.

Wall-eyed Drunk.

Wallop Potent alcoholic content or reaction.

Wallpapered Drunk.

Warmer Liquor.

Warmer-Upper Liquor.

Wash Inferior liquor.

Wash One's Ivories To take a drink.

Wash Still First still used when double distilling alcohol.

Wassail 1. Liquor. 2. Party at which a lot of alcohol is consumed.

Wassailed Drunk.

Wassailed-out Drunk.

Wassailed-up Drunk.

Wassailer Drunkard.

Waste A bar.

Wasted Drunk.

Water-betwitched Drink that has been watered down.

Water Bottle Abstainer.

Water Cart, On the Drunk.

Water of Life Alcohol.

Water-soaked Drunk.

Water Wagon, Fall off the To drink after trying to remain abstinent.

Water Wagon, On the *Same as* On the Wagon.

Watered Drunk.

Waterlogged Drunk.

Wattle To drink; from "What'll you have?"

Waxed Drunk.

Waxer Liquor.

Way, Out of the Drunk.

Weak-jointed Drunk.

Weary Drunk.

Weaving Drunk.

Weed Monkey Truck used to transport moonshine.

Weed Mule *Same as* Weed Monkey.

Weekend drinker One who drinks a lot during weekends but rarely during the rest of the week.

Well Away Drunk.

Well-bottled Drunk.

Well-fixed Drunk.

Well-heeled Drunk.

Well-jointed Drunk.

Well-lathered Drunk.

Well-lit Drunk.

Well-lubricated Drunk.

Well-mulled Drunk.

Well-oiled Very drunk.

Well-organized Drunk.

Well-primed Drunk.

Well-soaked Drunk.

Well-sprung Drunk.

Wernicke's Syndrome Pathological condition associated with chronic alcoholism. Symptoms include disorientation, muscle weakness, visual impairment, and other physical and mental problems.

Wester Drunkard.

Wet 1. Drunk. 2. A drink. 3. Political position opposed to prohibition.

Wet as the Atlantic Ocean Anti-prohibitionist.

Wet Both Eyes To drink until drunk.

Wet-brained Suffering from Wernicke's Syndrome.

Wet Canteen Store area where liquor can be bought.

Wet County County in which sale of beverage alcohol is legal.

Wet-Dry Advocate of prohibition who himself uses liquor.

Wet Enough for Rubber Boots Anti-prohibitionist.

Wet Goods Liquor.

Wet-handed Drunk.

Wet Muck Anti-prohibitionist.

Wet Night Night of hard drinking.

Wet Parson Clergyman who sometimes becomes drunk.

Wet Quaker One who pretends not to drink but does.

Wet Ship Ship on which the captain and crew drink excessively.

Wet Smack A drink.

Wet Spot A bar.

Wet Stuff Liquor.

Wet Subject One who is drunk.

Wet the Clay To take a drink.

Wet the other Eye To take a drink.

Wet the Sickle To take a drink.

Wet Your Whistle To take a drink.

Wetster A drunkard.

Wetter Anti-prohibitionist.

Wetting Drinking.

Wettish 1. Drunk. 2. Anti-prohibitionist.

Whacked-out Drunk.

Whale Heavy drinker.

Wham Alcoholic content or reaction.

Whammy Delirium Tremens.

What do you say? Invitation to drink.

What goes with it? Liquor.

What it takes Dash of liquor.

What will you liq? What would you like to drink?

What'll you have? What would you like to drink?

What-nosed Drunk.

What's the good news? What would you like to drink?

What's your medicine? What are you drinking?

Whazood Drunk.

Wheat Whiskey Alcohol beverage made from wheat grain.

Whet Morning drink.

Whiffled Drunk.

Whip-belly Vengeance *Same as* Whistle-belly Vengeance.

Whip Off To drink the entire contents of a glass without pausing.

Whipcat Drunk.

Whipped 1. Drunk. 2. *Same as* Whip Off.

Whipsey Drunk.

Whiskey Liquor made from cereal grains, usually containing over 50 percent alcohol.

Whiskey, Blended Mixture containing at least 20 percent pure whiskey, neutral spirits, other whiskeys, and flavorings.

Whiskey, Bonded Whiskey stored for at least four years in wood barrels and bottled at 100 proof. Does not contain blended whiskey.

Whiskey, Bourbon Whiskey distilled at less than 160 proof from fermented mash containing at least 51 percent corn. Must be stored at 125 proof or less in charred new oak barrels.

Whiskey, Corn Same as bourbon whiskey except mash must contain no less than 80 percent corn grain. Cannot be treated in any way with charred wood.

Whiskey, Light Whiskey distilled at less than 160 proof and stored in uncharred oak barrels.

Whiskey, Rye Same as bourbon except produced from mash containing at least 51 percent rye.

Whiskey, straight 1. Whiskey stored in new oak containers for at least two years. 2. Whiskey directly from the bottle.

Whiskey Bloat One bloated from drinking too much whiskey.

Whiskey Bottle A drunkard.

Whiskey Frisky Drunk on whiskey.

Whiskey Legger Bootlegger.

Whiskey Mill A bar.

Whiskey Nose Red swollen nose due to broken blood vessels caused by excessive drinking.

Whiskey Raddled Drunk on whiskey.

Whiskey Shot Drunk on whiskey.

Whiskey Skin Mixed drink made with whiskey.

Whiskey Smash *Same as* Whiskey Skin.

Whiskey Sodden Drunk on whiskey.

Whiskeyfied Drunk on whiskey.

Whiskied Drunk on whiskey.

Whiskin Flask containing liquor.

Whisper Illegal drinking place.

Whisper Joint *Same as* Whisper.

Whisperlow *Same as* Whisper.

Whistle Drunk Drunk.

Whistle Jacket Inferior beer.

Whistle Wetter Liquor.

Whistle-belly 1. Thin drink. 2. Sour or acid beer.

Whistle-belly Vengeance Popular alcohol drink in Massachusetts during colonial era. Made with sour beer, molasses, and brown bread crumbs.

White 1. Gin. 2. Liquor.

White Coffee Illegally sold whiskey.

White Coffer Whiskey.

White Eye Whiskey.

White Horse Whiskey.

White Lighting Illegally manufactured whiskey, colorless and made from corn. Usually with high alcohol content.

White Line Liquor diluted with water.

White Liner Alcoholic.

White Mule *Same as* White Lightning.

White Stuff Liquor.

White Tape Gin.

White Velvet Gin.

White Vinegar Cheap white wine.

White Wash Liquor.

White Wine Gin.

Whittled Drunk.

Who Shot John Potent moonshine whiskey.

Wholesaler One who buys whiskey from a Moonshiner and sells it to a Bootlegger.

Whoofits Hungover.

Whoop it up To go on a drinking spree.

Whooper-Up Liquor.

Whoopie Water 1. Liquor. 2. Champagne.

Whoops and Jingles Delirium Tremens.

Whoop-t-do Drinking spree.

Whooshed Drunk.

Whoozy Drunk.

Whoppin' the Cap Striking the top part of the moonshiner's still to determine the amount of pressure that has developed.

Wibble Bad liquor.

Wiffsniffer Prohibitionist.

Wilch Sediment or lees of beer or homemade wine.

Wild Cat Illicit liquor.

Wild Geronimo Mixture of barbiturates and alcohol.

Wildcatter *Same as* Moonshiner.

Wild-wave jockey Rum runner.

Willy-wacht Drink before going to bed.

Wilted Drunk.

Wind Wine.

Wine 1. Alcoholic beverage usually made from fermented grape juice. 2. Party at which the main beverage is wine.

Wine cellar Area of home or winery where wine is stored.

Wine Cooler Mixture of port wine and ginger ale.

Wine glass Special glass for serving wine, usually with stem and broad base.

Wine Nose Red nose due to broken blood vessels caused by frequent and excessive wine drinking.

Wine of the Poor Gin.

Wine-potted Drunk.

Wine Shits Diarrhea from drinking too much wine.

Wine Whooper Wine party.

Wined Up Drunk on wine.

Winefest Wine party.

Winery Business that makes wine.

Winey Drunk on wine.

Wingding A drinking spree.

Wing-heavy Drunk.

Wino Drunkard who primarily drinks wine.

Wino, Good-for-nothing Drunkard with no redeeming characteristics.

Winterized Drunk.

Wipe off your chin Invitation to drink.

Wiped Drunk.

Wiped Out Drunk.

Wired Drunk.

Wise Drunk.

Wish-Wash Weak, inferior liquor.

Witch Piss Poor quality liquor.

With a Breath On Drunk.

With an Affectionate Jag on Feeling libidinous as a result of drinking.

Withdrawal Various physical and psychological effects associated with cessation from chronic alcohol use. Physical reactions include convulsions, sweating, and fever. Psychological reactions include hallucinations, delusions, and tremors.

Without a Kick Not containing alcohol.

Without a Shirt Undiluted liquor.

Wobble Shop Place where beer is sold without a license.

Wobbly Drunk.

Woggled Drunk.

Woggly Drunk.

Women's Christian Temperance Union (WCTU) Organization started in 1874 to close saloons and increase public morality.

Wood alcohol Methanol. Poisonous fluid chemically related to alcohol; made by wood distillation. Sometimes consumed by skid row alcoholics when unable to get alcohol.

Woofle Water Liquor.

Woofled Drunk.

Wooshed Drunk.

Woozy Drunk.

Work the Can To drink considerable amounts of canned beer.

Worker Robber of intoxicated persons.

Worm Water-cooled pipe coil which causes heated alcohol vapors to condense in distillation.

Worm Box Water container in which the worm is submerged.

Wormwood Plant once used to make absinthe.

Wort Product resulting from infusion of barley into water. The second stage in making beer.

Wreath of Grog Blossoms Face full of pimples as a result of too much drinking.

Wrecked Drunk.

W/v "Weight by volume." The amount of alcohol in grams in a given volume of solution, usually 100 milliliters.

Y

Yadnarb Brandy.

Yappy Drunk.

Yard of Ale About a half-pint of ale, usually served in a glass with a wide bottom and narrow neck.

Yard of Flannel Pitcher-full of Flip in contrast to the large glass tumbler in which the drink was usually served.

Yaupish Drunk.

Years of the Big Thirst Prohibition era.

Yeast Single-celled organism which acts as a catalyst in turning sugar in fruit or grain into alcohol.

Yellowstone Water Weak, inferior liquor.

You Do Me Proud Acceptance of an offer to drink.

Z

Zagged Drunk.

Zapped Drunk.

Zig Zag Drunk.

Zig-zagged Drunk.

Zing Alcoholic content or reaction.

Zings Delirium Tremens.

Zip Alcoholic content or reaction.

Zip Up To add liquor to another beverage.

Zipped Drunk.

Zissified Drunk.

Zizz Alcoholic content or reaction.

Zoned Drunk.

Zonked Very drunk.

Zorked Drunk.

Zozzled Drunk.

Zymase Enzyme in yeast that breaks down sugar into alcohol and carbon dioxide.

Zyme Fermentation.

Zymology Science of fermentation.

Zymurgy Chemistry of fermentation.

Zythepsary Brewery.

Bibliography

Adams, R. F. *Western Words*. Norman, Okla.: University of Oklahoma Press, 1968.

Bartlett, J. R. *Dictionary of Americanisms: A Glossary of Words and Phrases Usually Regarded as Peculiar to The United States*. Boston: Little, Brown, and Co., 1896.

Berry, L. V., and M. Van Den Bark. *The American Thesaurus of Slang*. New York: T. Crowell, 1942.

Botkin, B. A. *New York City Folklore*. New York: Random House, 1956.

Brewer, T. *Brewer's Dictionary Of Phrase and Fable*. New York: Harper and Brothers, 1959.

Brophy, J., and E. Partridge. *Songs And Slang Of The British Soldier: 1914–1918*. London: Eric Partridge, 1930.

Brown, J. H. *Early American Beverages*. Rutland, Vt.: C. E. Tuttle, Co., 1966.

Burke, J. P. "The Argot of the Racketeers." *American Mercury* 27 (1930), 454–458.

Carr, J. *The Second Oldest Profession. An Informal History of Moonshining in America*. Englewood Cliffs, N. J.: Prentice-Hall, 1972.

Carson, G. *The Social History of Bourbon*. New York: Dodd, Mead and Co., 1963.

Ciardi, J. *A Browser's Dictionary And Native's Guide To The Unknown American Language*. New York: Harper and Row, 1980.

Farmer, J. S., and W. E. Henley. *Slang And Its Analogues*. 1890–1904. Reprint. New York: Arno Press, 1970.

Flexner, S. B. *I Hear America Talking: An Illustrated Treasury of American Words and Phrases*. New York: Van Nostrand Reinhold, 1976.

Fox, R. K. *The Slang Dictionary of New York, London, and Paris*. New York: National Police Gazette, 1880.

Fraser, E., and J. Gibbons. *Soldier And Sailor Words And Phrases*. London: George Routledge and Sons, 1925.

Funk, C. E. *Heavens to Betsy!* New York: Harper and Row, 1955.

Gent, B. E. *A New Dictionary of the Terms Ancient and Modern of the Canting Crew, in its Several Tribes, of Gypsies, Beggars, Thieves, Cheats, etc.*

with an Addition of Some Proverbs, Phrases, Figurative Speeches, etc. London: W. Hawes, 1899.

Granville, J. *Sea Slang of the 20th Century.* London: Winchester Publications, 1949.

Grose, F. *A Classical Dictionary of the Vulgar Tongue.* N.p. 1788.

Hall, B. *Travels In North America.* 1829. Reprint. Graz, Austria: Akademische Druck u. Verlagsanstalt, 1965.

Hall, B. H. *A Collection of College Words And Customs.* Cambridge, Mass.: John Bartlett, 1856.

Hardin, A. "Volstead English." *American Speech* 7, (1931), 81–88.

Heywood, J. *The Proverbs, Epigrams, and Miscellanies of John Heywood.* 1562. Reprint. Guildford, England: Charles W. Traylen, 1966.

Larson, C. "The Drinkers Dictionary." *American Speech* 12, (1937), 87–92.

Levine, H. G. "The vocabulary of drunkenness." *Journal of Studies on Alcohol* 42 (1981) 1038–1051.

Maitland, J. *The American Slang Dictionary.* Chicago: R. J. Kittridge, 1891.

Marryat, F. *A Diary in America.* 1839. Reprint. New York: A. A. Knopf, 1962.

Maurer, D. W. "The Argot of the Moonshiner." *American Speech* 24, (1949), 3–13.

Mencken, H. L. *The American Language.* New York: A. A. Knopf, 1963.

Moor, E. *Suffolk Words and Phrases.* 1823. Reprint. New York: Augustus M. Kelley, 1970.

Morris, W., and M. Morris. *Dictionary of Word And Phrase Origins.* New York: Harper and Row, 1977.

Nares, R. *A Glossary; or, Collection Of Words, Phrases, Names, And Allusions To Customs, Proverbs, Etc., Which Have Been Thought To Require Illustration In The Works Of English Authors, Particularly Shakespeare And His Contemporaries.* Revised by Halliwell, J., and Wright, O. T., London: Reeves and Turner, Inc., 1888.

Partridge, E. *A Dictionary of Slang And Unconventional English.* New York: Macmillan and Co., 1974.

Potter, H. T. *A New Dictionary of All the Cant and Flash Languages, Both Ancient and Modern; Used by Gypsies, Beggars, Swindlers, Shoplifters, Peterers, Starrers, Footpads, Highway Men, Sharpers, and Every Class of Offenders, From a Lully Prigger to a High Tober Gloak.* London: W. MacIntosh, 1790.

Randolph, V. "Wet words in Kansas." *American Speech* 4, 1929, 385–389.

Rogers, B. *The Queen's Vernacular.* San Francisco: Straight Arrow Books, 1972.

Rubington, E. "The language of 'drunks'" *Quarterly Journal of Studies on Alcohol* 32, (1971), 721–740.

Shay, F. *A Sailor's Treasury.* New York: W. W. Norton, 1951.

Sheppard, H. *The Dictionary of Railway Slang.* New York: Dillington House, 1967.

Thornton, R. H. *An American Glossary.* Philadelphia: J. B. Lippincott, 1912.

Tucker, G. M. *American English.* New York: A. A. Knopf, 1921.

Walsh, W. S. *Hand-book of Literary Curiosities.* Philadelphia: J. P. Lippincott, 1892.

Ware, J. R. *Passing English Of The Victorian Era*. 1909. Reprint. New York: EP Publishing, 1972.

Weekley, E. *Words Ancient And Modern*. London: John Murray, 1946.

Weems, M. L. *The Drunkard's Looking Glass*. 1813. Reprint in Weems, M. L. *Three Discourses*. New York: Random House, 1929.

Wentworth, H. and S. B. Flexner. *Dictionary of American Slang*. New York: T. Crowell, 1960.

Weseen, M. H. *A Dictionary of American Slang*. New York: Thomas Y. Crowell Co., 1934.

About the Compiler

ERNEST L. ABEL is a Research Scientist at the Research Institute on Alcoholism in Buffalo, New York. His other works include *Lead and Reproduction* (1985), *A Dictionary of Drug Abuse Terms and Terminology* (1984), *Narcotics and Reproduction* (1983), *Drugs and Sex* (1983), *Alcohol and Reproduction* (1982), and *Smoking and Reproduction* (1982), all published by Greenwood Press.

www.ingramcontent.com/pod-product-compliance
Lightning Source LLC
Chambersburg PA
CBHW050228270326
41914CB00003BA/614